Dr. Sarah Brewer
natural
health
guru

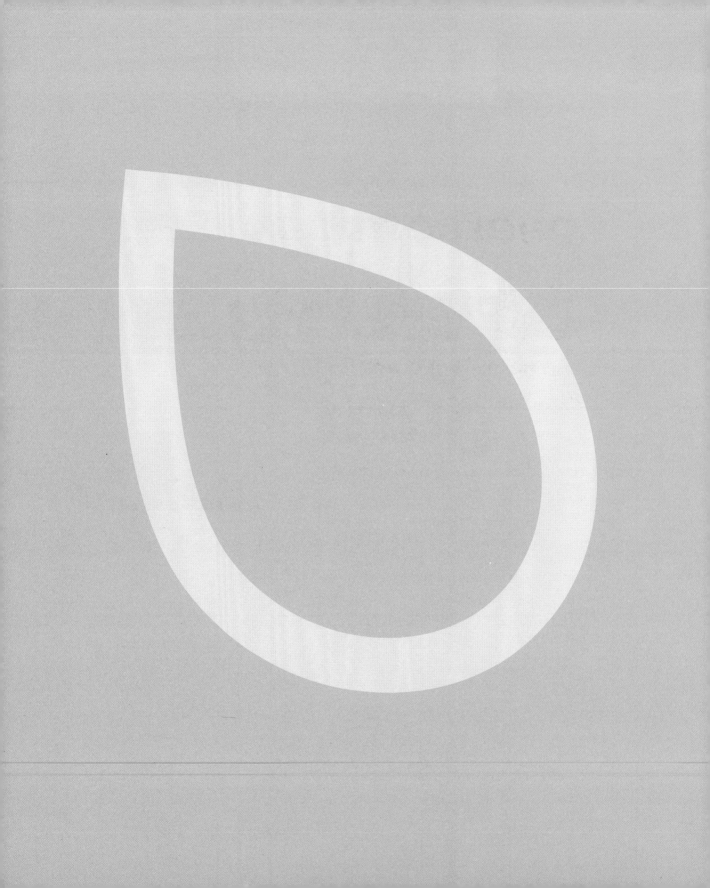

overcoming
arthritis
the complete complementary
health program

Dr. Sarah Brewer

In association with The Complementary Medical Association

DUNCAN BAIRD PUBLISHERS

LONDON

Natural Health Guru: Overcoming Arthritis
Dr. Sarah Brewer

For my wonderful husband, Richard

Distributed in the USA and Canada by
Sterling Publishing Co., Inc.
387 Park Avenue South
New York, NY 10016-8810

This edition first published in the UK and USA in 2009 by
Duncan Baird Publishers Ltd.
Sixth Floor, Castle House
75–76 Wells Street
London W1T 3QH

Managing Editor: Grace Cheetham
Editor: Kesta Desmond
Managing Designer: Manisha Patel
Designer: Gail Jones
Commissioned artwork: Mark Watkinson
Commissioned photography: Toby Scott and Simon Smith
Styling: Mari Mererid Willliams
Picture research: Susannah Stone

Library of Congress Cataloging-in-Publication Data available

ISBN: 978-1-84483-728-1
10 9 8 7 6 5 4 3 2 1

Typeset in Univers
Color reproduction by Scanhouse, Malaysia
Printed in China by Imago

Publisher's note:
The information in this book is not intended as a substitute for
professional medical advice and treatment. If you are pregnant or
are suffering from any medical conditions or health problems, it is
recommended that you consult a medical professional before following
any of the advice or practices suggested in this book. Duncan Baird
Publishers, or any other persons who have been involved in working
on this publication, cannot accept responsibility for any injuries
or damage incurred as a result of following the information, exercises,
or therapeutic techniques contained in this book.

Notes on the recipes
Unless otherwise stated: use large eggs, and medium fruit and
vegetables. Use fresh ingredients, including herbs. All-purpose and
wholewheat flours should be scooped with the cup measure and then
the surface leveled. 1tsp. = 5ml, 1tbsp. = 15ml, 1 cup = 240ml

For information about custom editions, special sales, premium
and corporate purchases, please contact Sterling Special Sales
Department at 800-805-5489 or specialsales@sterlingpub.com.

contents

arthritis
introduction

Arthritis is the inflammation of one or more joints and it comes in a variety of forms. All cause similar symptoms of pain, swelling, stiffness, and restriction of movement, which can have a major effect on quality of life. Worldwide, as many as one in two people over the age of 60 have self-reported arthritis symptoms. These symptoms can be mild and intermittent or they can be severe and continuous. In the United States alone, an estimated 40 million people have arthritis, and the number is expected to reach 59 million by 2020.

Although it becomes more common with advancing age, joint problems affect younger people, too. An estimated 25 people in a thousand under the age of 40 have arthritis, with juvenile arthritis affecting between one and four out of every thousand children in different countries.

Follow your doctor's advice
The information and advice given in this book is for general information only. It's not intended to replace individual advice from your own doctor. My approach is holistic and designed to complement the treatments your doctor prescribes. If you follow one or more of the programs in Part Three, please treat my advice as a guide only and always follow the advice of your doctor or other healthcare professionals who know your specific needs in detail. In particular, never stop taking your arthritis medication, except under the advice and supervision of your own doctor.

The good news is that many cases of arthritis can be relieved, postponed, or even prevented by good joint care—that's my aim in writing this book. Many of us tend to take our joints for granted until we start to experience pain or discomfort. But by the time you notice symptoms significant damage might already have occurred. The sooner you start looking after your joints, the better. If any of the following points apply to you, I recommend you start to make diet and lifestyle changes now:

- You are aged 40 or over.
- Arthritis runs in your family.
- You are overweight.
- You do little regular exercise.
- Your work involves repetitive movements of one or more joints.
- You feel the need to stretch your back every day.
- You notice creakiness in one or more joints.
- You notice that a joint, such as your knee or hip, is less flexible than before, or you find it difficult to straighten a joint fully.
- You can no longer touch your toes when standing with your knees straight.
- You have limited neck rotation and can no longer align your chin with your shoulder tip, or are unable to touch the front of your chest with your chin.
- Your joints are swelling or changing shape.
- Your fingers and toes increasingly tend to get cold and stiff.
- A joint starts aching, especially after exercise.
- Your knees are painful when you kneel or sit on them.

Many people with joint pain avoid exercise but, as discussed on pages 66–69, regular exercise is vitally important for long-term joint health. If you have arthritis, it's important you don't give up an active life in favor of rest. Although your joints need *some* rest, too much will make your muscles weak and increase your joint stiffness. Simple exercises, such as stretching, walking, cycling, or swimming, can go a long way to keep your joints healthy and flexible. If you're overweight, your weight-bearing joints will have to work harder than they would otherwise. (I explain how you can lose weight on pages 70–71.)

Like your heart, your joints thrive best on a healthy lifestyle and a diet that is rich in superfoods (see pages 54–57). In Part Three, I show you how you can change your lifestyle and diet for maximum benefit. Because everyone is different and no diet and lifestyle plan will suit all individuals, I've created three different approaches: a gentle, a moderate, and a full-strength program. To help you work out which one is right for you, complete the questionnaire on pages 75–76.

For many people, the gentle program is a good place to start. It introduces you to healthy eating principles, such as eating more fruit, vegetables, and fish. I suggest you take food supplements, such as glucosamine, at a dose that will have a significant, beneficial effect on your arthritis symptoms. I also show you some useful stretch exercises, and introduce you to complementary health approaches, such as aromatherapy and homeopathy. A month on the gentle program can significantly reduce the level of inflammation in your joints.

If your responses to the questionnaire suggest that you have a sensitivity to plants of the nightshade family, such as tomatoes, bell peppers, chilies, eggplants, and potatoes, the moderate program shows you how to exclude these foods from your diet. I also provide some stretch and range-of-movement

exercises, and introduce you to complementary approaches, such as reflexology and meditation. If you're sensitive to foods from the nightshade family, your symptoms should become less troublesome within a month of following the moderate program.

For people whose questionnaire identifies a pronounced inflammatory component to their arthritis, the full-strength program will provide an eating plan that significantly increases your daily intake of antioxidants and spices with a natural, analgesic action. I also include an exercise program that will help you stay active and flexible; and I introduce you to complementary techniques, such as acupressure and acupuncture. If your arthritis is linked with inflammatory reactions within your joints, the full-strength program has the potential to relieve symptoms within a month.

I've created a website to accompany the Natural Health Guru series of books. Please visit www. naturalhealthguru.co.uk regularly to tell me how you get on with the programs, to post your successes, and to read the latest information and research.

Look out for these symbols

Throughout this book I have included boxes that highlight useful, interesting, or important pieces of information. Each box bears a symbol (see below). The arrow symbol indicates a box that contains practical instructions. The plus sign means the box contains additional information about the subject being discussed or about asthma in general. The exclamation mark indicates a warning or a caution.

Understanding arthritis

A condition that appears in many guises, arthritis can take the form of **osteoarthritis**, which is linked to increasing age, and wear and tear on the joints; or it can be a condition, such as **rheumatoid arthritis** and **psoriatic arthropathy** in which the body's own immune system attacks the joints. **Gout** is another type of arthritis. Whichever type you have, the **underlying symptoms** are essentially the same—joint pain, stiffness, swelling, and restricted movement. To help you understand the nature of arthritis I describe the **different types of joint in the human body** and the different types of arthritis that can affect them. Although the causes of arthritis are not yet fully understood, I explain the **current understanding of the genetics** that underlie autoimmune arthritis, and the factors that can damage joints and lead to osteoarthritis. Your doctor will diagnose which type of arthritis you have using a range of techniques, such as physical examination, x-rays, and analysis of your joint fluid. A number of **diagnostic blood tests** are also available. I explain the variety of painkilling and immune-modifying drugs that can help control your symptoms. I also describe the variety of different approaches **orthopedic surgery** can offer.

what is arthritis?

The word arthritis literally means inflammation of a joint. A joint forms where two bones come into close contact with each other. Some joints have limited flexibility and are designed to allow for growth, such as those in the skull which fuse together to form suture joints only after the skull is fully mature. Other joints have a limited amount of movement to absorb shock, and are stabilized by pads of cartilage, such as those between the two long bones in your lower leg (the tibia and fibula). Most joints, however, can move more freely through a variable range of movements. To fully understand what happens when arthritis develops, it's useful to have an understanding of the joints and their surrounding structures.

Understanding your joints

There are six different types of moveable joint, all of which can be affected by arthritis.

In a ball-and-socket joint, a round-shaped bone surface fits inside a cup-shaped socket in another bone. This type of joint, such as the hip, has the greatest range of movement. The shoulder ball-and-socket joint has the widest range of movement of all. It's known as a multiaxial joint, as the arm can move in more than two planes: up and down, backward and forward, plus rotating in a circle at the side of the body.

Ellipsoid joints consist of an oval-shaped bone surface fitting into an oval-shaped cup in another bone. This type of joint, such as the wrist, can move back and forth or from side to side, but full rotation is limited.

In a saddle joint, two U-shaped bone surfaces fit together at right angles to rock back and forth and from side to side. This joint gives the thumb limited rotation.

Hinge joints consist of the cylindrical surface of one bone sitting inside the curve of another. A hinge joint, such as that of the fingers, allows movement in one plane. The elbow and knee are modified hinge joints.

In a pivot joint, one bone swivels inside a space formed by another bone. The pivot joint between two upper neck vertebrae (the axis and atlas) allows the head to swivel from side to side.

Finally, in a gliding joint, two joint surfaces that are almost flat move by sliding over each other. Some of the joints in the vertebral column, hands and feet are of this kind, and are bound together by strong ligaments that limit their range of movement.

Your joints are made of other elements, too:

Ligaments Joints are bound together by tough, slightly elastic bands of collagen fiber known as ligaments. These form a capsule around a mobile joint and provide reinforcement. Some joints, such as the knee, also have internal ligaments for additional stability, allowing the joint to bend while stopping the ends of the bones from moving back and forth, or side to side. People described as "double-jointed" have a wider range of joint movement than usual as a result of inheriting looser, more elastic ligaments (known as hyperlaxity).

Cartilage This slippery substance protects the surfaces of mobile joints from wear and tear by allowing the bones to slide easily over one another. Disks of cartilage are found in the knee joint and where the jaw bone articulates (forms a joint) with the skull. These disks of articular cartilage act like washers

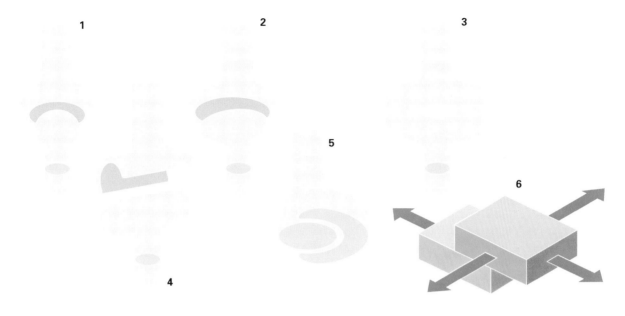

The six types of joint in the body
1. Ball and socket (hip); 2. Ellipsoid (wrist); 3. Saddle (thumb); 4. Hinge (elbow); 5. Pivot (upper neck); 6. Gliding (some joints in the spine, hands, and feet)

to reduce friction between moving bones. Cartilage contains collagen and elastin fibers, plus a tough, gel-like substance, called the matrix, which is secreted by embedded cells called chondrocytes.

Synovial fluid The capsule of a mobile joint is lined with a thin tissue called the synovial membrane. This secretes a thick, slippery fluid that resembles egg white. Synovial fluid cushions and oils the joints, provides them with nutrients and reduces friction between the articular cartilage.

Tendons Joints are moved by the relaxation and contraction of opposing groups of muscle, which attach to the bones via elastic strands of tissue known as tendons. The tendons run within oiled tubes, known as sheaths.

Bursas These are fluid-filled sacs above and below certain joints, such as the knee. They store synovial fluid, and act as cushions to prevent tendons and muscles from rubbing at pressure points.

Types of arthritis
There are many different types of arthritis—the most common type is osteoarthritis followed by rheumatoid arthritis.

Osteoarthritis (OA) This involves degeneration of the cartilage that protects the bone ends within a joint. Without cartilage protection, the bone ends rub together and become inflamed. As the cartilage becomes pitted, cracked, and flaky, synovial fluid leaks through the cracks into the underlying bone. The causes the bone to thicken and become mildly inflamed, forming small cysts and bony swellings called osteophytes. The bone ends might eventually rub together. The synovial membrane and joint capsule also thicken and the space inside the joint becomes increasingly narrow. As a result of all these processes, joint movements become painful, stiff, and restricted, and affected joints can change in appearance—they might start to look knobbly and enlarged. Walking awkwardly causes associated ligaments and muscles to ache, and joint pain often keeps you awake at night. You can feel or hear creaking and cracking as you move, and your muscles can become wasted from lack of use. Osteoarthritis usually affects larger, weight-bearing joints such as the hips, knees, and lower spine, but it can also affect other mobile joints, such as the neck, shoulders, elbows, wrists, ankles, fingers, toes, and jaw.

Joints affected by arthritis

Osteoarthritis begins with a deterioration in the cartilage in your joints. This is usually followed by damage to the bone and synovial membrane. Rheumatoid arthritis begins with the inflammation of the synovial membrane, followed by cartilage and bone destruction.

Rheumatoid arthritis This develops when your immune system wrongly identifies parts of a joint as "foreign" and attacks them. The synovial membrane lining certain joints becomes inflamed because of abnormal activity of certain immune cells (T and B lymphocytes). Inflammation gradually spreads from the synovial membrane to the tendon sheaths, and the membrane lining the bursas (see page 11) around affected joints. Eventually, the bone can be affected, too, to cause characteristic joint deformities, such as those in the hands, in which the fingers deviate toward the little finger. Rheumatoid arthritis usually affects the smaller joints in the wrists, hands, and feet, but can also occur in the neck, knees, and ankles. It usually develops symmetrically so the same joints on both sides of the body become red, hot, and swollen. Early morning stiffness that lasts for several hours is common, as are weight loss, fever, and exhaustion. Rheumatoid arthritis tends to be a remitting and relapsing disease in which flare-ups are followed by periods in which symptoms improve. The

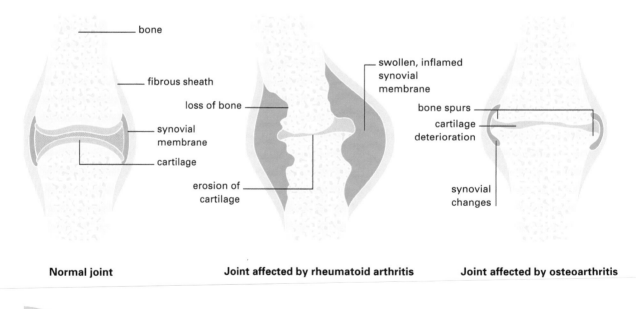

bone

fibrous sheath

loss of bone

synovial membrane

cartilage

erosion of cartilage

swollen, inflamed synovial membrane

bone spurs

cartilage deterioration

synovial changes

Normal joint   **Joint affected by rheumatoid arthritis**   **Joint affected by osteoarthritis**

understanding arthritis

autoimmune process can also attack other parts of the body, including the skin, muscles, blood vessels, heart, lungs, and eyes. Because of its widespread, systemic nature, people with rheumatoid arthritis are also more likely to experience a heart attack or stroke than others —probably because inflammation affects the circulation and thickens the blood, too. If you have rheumatoid arthritis, it's important to have regular cardiovascular checks. Children can also develop rheumatoid arthritis. When it develops under the age of 16, it is known as juvenile rheumatoid arthritis or Still's disease.

Other types of arthritis Joint inflammation can be the result of autoimmune disease, such as psoriasis, lupus, and inflammatory bowel disease, as well as the following:

- Gout—a form of arthritis in which needlelike crystals of a substance called uric acid are deposited in a joint, typically at the base of the big toe. It can also affect other small joints in the feet and hands, especially the thumb, as well as larger joints, such as the knee, ankle, or wrist. Uric acid crystals cause severe inflammation and exquisite tenderness with redness and swelling of the affected joint. Mild fever can also occur.
- Pseudogout—this is similar to gout, but calcium pyrophosphate, rather than uric acid, is deposited within a joint, most often the knee, although also the wrist, shoulder, ankle, elbow, and hand.
- Septic arthritis—this is when a joint is infected by bacteria, a virus, or even certain fungi. Most cases involve the skin bacteria *Staphylococcus aureus*.
- Reactive arthritis—this results from infections that do not directly involve the joint. It's also known as postexposure arthritis, and it occurs when antibodies made to fight an infection in one part of the body attack the joints as if they were also

infected, when they are not. This form of immune attack most commonly affects people who carry a gene known as human lymphocyte antigen B27 (HLA-B27). Reactive arthritis can occur following gastroenteritis (food poisoning) with organisms such as salmonella, campylobacter, clostridium, shigella, and *Entamoeba histolytica*. It can also follow genitourinary infections such as chlamydia or gonorrhea. Lyme disease is also more likely to cause reactive arthritis than septic arthritis.

- Ankylosing spondylitis—also more common in people carrying the HLA-B27 gene, this is a form of autoimmune disease in which inflammation affects the sacroiliac joints in the pelvis, and small joints within the vertebral column that can eventually fuse. It can also affect the hips, knees, and shoulders. Other symptoms include loss of appetite, tiredness, feeling unwell, and inflammation of the iris in the eye (iritis).
- Psoriatic arthropathy—this is a form of autoimmune arthritis that affects between 10 and 20 percent of people with psoriasis (an inflammatory skin disease). There's no link between the severity of skin symptoms and whether or not your joints are affected. As with other forms of autoimmune arthritis, the synovial membrane becomes inflamed and releases more fluid than normal, and the joint becomes tender and swollen. As inflammation continues, it spreads to the cartilage underneath and can eventually erode the bone. As the tendons are lined and lubricated by a synovial membrane, these also become inflamed, especially around the elbows, wrists, and heels. The most common type of psoriatic arthropathy involves the small joints of the fingers and toes, producing sausage-shaped digits. Pitting of the nails and inflammation of the sacroiliac joints in the pelvis are also common.

causes, signs, and symptoms

Although there are many different types of arthritis, with many different underlying causes, the basic symptoms and signs of joint damage are similar in every case.

Why arthritis develops

The reasons why some people develop arthritis while others don't is not fully understood, but is believed to result from interactions between a number of factors, including heredity, lifestyle, and environment.

Genes All types of arthritis appear to run in families and are likely to involve certain genes. For example, it makes sense that if you inherit a weaker or thinner layer of articular cartilage (see pages 10–11), you're likely to be more prone to osteoarthritis. And genetic mutation affecting collagen production has been linked with the premature breakdown of joint cartilage in some families. Researchers have also found that genes that affect communication between cartilage-making cells (chondrocytes) influence your susceptibility for developing osteoarthritis of the hip. Overall, it's thought that 60 percent of osteoarthritis has a genetic basis, and 25 percent of cases result from a single, specific, gene mutation.

One of the strongest hereditary links with arthritis involves the gene HLA-B27, which codes for a specific protein on the surfaces of white blood cells. If you inherit this gene, you're four times more likely than normal to develop reactive arthritis, psoriatic arthropathy, or ankylosing spondylitis. But, although 90 percent of people with ankylosing spondylitis carry the HLA-B27 gene, only a fraction (between two

and six percent) of those who possess HLA-B27 go on to develop ankylosing spondylitis. This suggests another trigger is needed; for example, inheriting other associated genes, or exposure to an environmental trigger, such as a specific infection.

Researchers have found that inheriting another gene involved in cell "self" recognition, called HLA-DR4, significantly increases the risk of developing rheumatoid arthritis, psoriatic arthritis, and reactive arthritis following Lyme disease.

Among identical twins, if one twin develops an autoimmune type of arthritis, such as rheumatoid arthritis, the chance the other twin will develop it is only 15 to 30 percent, suggesting nongenetic factors, such as exposure to a virus, are necessary for the disease to express itself. Twenty percent of people with gout have a family history of the disease.

Infection A joint damaged by direct infection (septic arthritis) is likely to develop osteoarthritis in the future. Infection can also trigger autoimmune arthritis in some people. For example, people with rheumatoid arthritis appear to have higher levels of antibodies against the Epstein-Barr virus than people without.

Gender Women are five times more likely to develop rheumatoid arthritis than men, but men are three times more likely to develop ankylosing spondylitis than women, and to have it more severely. This suggests that some forms of arthritis have causes that are sex-linked (perhaps carried on the X or Y chromosomes that determine sex) or are in some way affected by male or female hormones (testosterone or estrogen).

For example, gout is nine times more common in men than women, because estrogen promotes the excretion of uric acid crystals into urine.

Age Osteoarthritis usually develops over many years, and becomes more common with increasing age. This is probably because the water content of cartilage decreases with age, and it becomes more brittle and less easy to repair. Most over-65s have osteoarthritis in at least one joint, although only 30 percent of those with x-ray evidence of osteoarthritis have pain at the relevant site. Autoimmune diseases also tend to start at specific times of life. For example, ankylosing spondylitis tends to develop between 16 and 30 years of age, and seldom in people over the age of 40. Similarly, a quarter of people with rheumatoid arthritis develop symptoms before the age of 30, and most new cases occur in the 40 to 50 age group. And in four out of five children with juvenile rheumatoid arthritis, symptoms disappear before the age of 20. Age is undoubtedly implicated in the cause of arthritis, but many centenarians have retained healthy, pain-free joints, so arthritis needs other triggers too.

Excess weight Being overweight greatly increases the risk of osteoarthritis in weight-bearing joints. This is because joint damage is partly dependent on the load the joint has to support. As a result, someone who is overweight is seven times more likely to develop osteoarthritis of the knee than someone in the healthy weight range for their height.

Previous joint damage People who put excessive strain on their joints in early life (for example, athletes), or those who have previously injured their joints through accidents or sport, are at increased risk of developing osteoarthritis in later life. A joint previously damaged by septic arthritis or recurrent episodes of gout is also likely to progress to osteoarthritis, as a result of irregularities on the surface of cartilage.

What are the symptoms?

The main signs and symptoms of arthritis are localized pain, tenderness, redness, hotness, swelling, stiffness, and loss of movement. These can be acute or chronic (long term). Acute joint inflammation resolves once the immediate cause is removed, such as the infecting organisms in the case of septic arthritis, or the crystals deposited in gout or pseudogout. Chronic inflammation occurs in osteoarthritis, where articular cartilage remains thin and brittle, and in autoimmune arthritis, where immune cells continue to misidentify the synovial membrane as foreign. Abnormal immune reactions also account for the tiredness and fatigue that typically accompany autoimmune diseases.

Why do joints get inflamed?
Inflammation is an important part of the body's healing process—it occurs when immune cells congregate to destroy tissues that are infected or diseased. When a patroling white blood cell enters a joint and identifies something as wrong, it secretes a number of chemical alarm signals known as cytokines. These attract other immune cells into the area and superstimulate them, so they are ready to fight infection or destroy damaged or abnormal body cells. Histamine is also released, which causes small blood vessels to dilate and become more permeable, bringing in blood and nutrients while flushing away toxins. The body also produces chemicals that stimulate pain receptors, which are nature's way of making you rest and immobilize a joint while healing occurs. All these reactions are responsible for the characteristic symptoms of an arthritis flare-up.

diagnosing arthritis

Your doctor will look at your joints and listen to a description of your symptoms as part of the diagnosis of arthritis. He or she is also likely to use x-rays, blood tests, and other investigative techniques to help to identify the cause of your joint pain.

Case history

Your doctor will ask you about your symptoms and which joints are affected. Morning stiffness that goes within 30 minutes, or stiffness that comes on later in the day after repetitive use, is usually a result of osteoarthritis, but morning stiffness that lasts longer than 30 minutes is more typical of rheumatoid arthritis. If nonsymmetrical joints are affected (for example,

one hip, one knee, one hand), then osteoarthritis is the most likely diagnosis, but if your joint symptoms are symmetrical (for example, both hands or wrists, both knees), this suggests rheumatoid arthritis, especially if your joints are red, swollen, warm, and tender.

Your doctor will also ask about any previous personal history relating to your joints, such as injury, and about your family history of arthritic conditions.

Physical examination

During an examination, a doctor will assess how red, swollen, and warm your joints are and whether there is a fluid buildup (effusion) within the joint. He or she will also look for the following:

- Bony or soft tissue nodules. Heberden's nodes and Bouchard's nodes are bony nodules that frequently develop around the joints of the fingers in older people with osteoarthritis, while people with rheumatoid arthritis develop rheumatoid nodules under the skin, especially at the elbow and down the forearm.
- The characteristic deformities of rheumatoid arthritis, such as boutonnière and swan-neck deformities of the fingers (see opposite), owing to erosion of finger joints, tendons, and ligaments. The fingers can also deviate toward the little finger owing to destruction of the knuckle joints.
- Marked muscle wasting (characteristic of rheumatoid arthritis).
- Swellings, called tophi, caused by a build up of uric acid crystals. They may erode through the skin in white, chalky nodules. Tophi are a sign of gout.

How many joints are affected?
The number of painful joints can be an indication of which type of arthritis you have. Pain that affects a single joint is known as monoarthritis. This is usually characteristic of osteoarthritis, trauma, infection (septic arthritis), or a crystalline arthritis (gout or pseudogout). Pain involving two, three, or four joints is called oligoarthritis and suggests either osteoarthritis or an autoimmune condition such as rheumatoid arthritis or psoriatic arthropathy. Pain affecting five or more joints is referred to as polyarthritis. This is indicative of a widespread, autoimmune disorder, such as rheumatoid arthritis, psoriatic arthritis, or joint involvement in another autoimmune condition, such as lupus (an ulcerative skin disease).

- Pinprick depressions in the fingernails, called pitting, are a sign of psoriatic arthropathy.
- Limited movement in any of the joints.
- "Crunching" or an audible sound when you move a joint.

X-rays

If you have osteoarthritis, x-rays of the affected joint can show a characteristic narrowing and irregularity of the joint space, as well as bone changes, such as increased density in the bone ends, formation of bony lumps (osteophytes), and "holes" in the bone beneath the cartilage, known as pseudocysts. Lack of these findings, however, does not exclude osteoarthritis. Similarly, some people can have x-ray findings consistent with osteoarthritis, but have no symptoms or disability.

What is arthrocentesis?

When a single joint is inflamed and swollen, a doctor might take a sample of the joint fluid using a sterile needle and syringe under local anesthetic. Normal joint fluid is slightly sticky (viscous) and is either crystal clear or a light straw color. If the fluid is cloudy, this is a sign of inflammation. If there is obvious pus in the fluid, this suggests septic arthritis. Analysis of joint fluid can detect the presence of protein, white blood cells, red blood cells, bacteria, and crystals. If the joint fluid forms a clot within one hour of collection, this shows the presence of a clotting protein fibrin, and is characteristic of inflammation of the synovial membrane.

How arthritis affects the finger joints

Sometimes the appearance of your joints is sufficient to diagnose arthritis. For example, bony nodules at the finger joints can be a sign of osteoarthritis; and finger deformities can be a sign of rheumatoid arthritis.

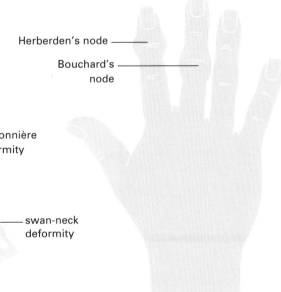

Herberden's node

Bouchard's node

boutonnière deformity

swan-neck deformity

Hand affected by rheumatoid arthritis

Hand affected by osteoarthritis

Laboratory tests

Laboratory tests can help differentiate between different types of arthritis, and can also help monitor disease activity and the effectiveness of treatment once a diagnosis is established.

Full blood count This gives a complete analysis of the white blood cells, red blood cells, platelets (clotting cell fragments), and the amount of red blood pigment (hemoglobin) present in your blood. A raised white-blood-cell level suggests that an active infection is present; low levels of white blood cells, red blood cells, and hemoglobin suggest you might have a chronic inflammatory disease, such as rheumatoid arthritis.

Erythrocyte sedimentation rate (ESR) This measures how quickly your red blood cells clump together and fall down a glass column. ESR is measured in millimetres per hour. A level above 100 mm/hr is an indication of abnormal inflammation that is usually autoimmune or infective in nature.

C-reactive protein (CRP) This is a "sticky" protein produced by the liver as part of the body's inflammatory response. Your CRP level is a more sensitive marker of inflammation than ESR, so doctors are increasingly using this test. Levels of 3 mg/L or higher are considered raised.

Antibody blood tests A raised level of antibodies suggests an infection or an autoimmune response.

Antinuclear antibodies (ANA) These are abnormal autoantibodies aimed against parts of the nucleus found in the middlle of all body cells, except red blood cells. Medium to high antinuclear antibody levels suggest an autoimmune disease, and are found in 30 to 50 percent of people with rheumatoid arthritis.

Rheumatoid factor (RF) This is an antibody found in around 80 percent of people with rheumatoid arthritis and about one percent of healthy people without rheumatoid arthritis. It is not fully diagnostic, however, because RF is also found in some people with other autoimmune conditions, such as lupus; in people with long-term viral infections, such as chronic hepatitis; and in some people with leukemia.

Anti-cyclic citrullinated peptide (anti-CCP) This is an antibody aimed against an unusual amino acid called citrulline. Chains of amino acids that include citrulline are found in joints affected by rheumatoid arthritis, but not other forms of arthritis. Its presence means there is a 95 percent chance you have rheumatoid arthritis.

HLA-tissue typing Some types of autoimmune arthritis are more likely in people with certain genes such as HLA-B27 and HLA-DR4 (see page 14). If your joint symptoms are difficult to diagnose, it can help to know whether or not you carry these genes.

Uric acid level If gout is suspected, a high level of uric acid in the blood helps to confirm the diagnosis.

Other tests

You might need a range of other tests during the diagnosis of an inflamed joint, including computed axial tomography (CAT) or magnetic resonance imaging (MRI) scans. These produce detailed, crosssectional images of the internal structures of a joint. Arthroscopy, in which a small optic tube (arthroscope) is inserted into the joint under general anesthetic, also allows direct viewing of the joint to evaluate degenerative changes and to determine the cause of pain and inflammation. A relatively new procedure, thermal imaging, can show the degree of inflammation by measuring changes in temperature across the joints.

treating arthritis

The medical treatment of all types of arthritis initially involves painkillers, such as paracetamol, and nonsteroidal anti-inflammatory drugs (NSAIDs), such as ibuprofen. You might also be offered physiotherapy. In addition, some forms of arthritis require disease-modifying drugs that damp down abnormal immune reactions. If your joint symptoms aren't relieved by drug therapy and physiotherapy, you might need joint replacement surgery.

Painkillers

Pain is a subjective, unpleasant sensation that's associated with actual or potential tissue damage. Because it's subjective, and can't be measured directly, your doctor relies heavily on your description of pain to select the right strength of drug. He or she might ask you to rate your pain on a scale of zero to 10: zero is no pain and 10 is the worst pain imaginable.

Paracetamol (acetaminophen) This the most widely used analgesic for arthritis, because it's effective against mild to moderate pain and has the least potential to cause adverse side effects when used at the correct dose of no more than 1 g, every four to six hours, up to a maximum dose of 4 g daily. Paracetamol has a direct effect on the brain to both kill pain and lower fever, but it doesn't have an anti-inflammatory action and doesn't reduce swelling or stiffness. It's, therefore, most helpful for osteoarthritis in which joint inflammation is minimal. Check with a doctor before taking paracetamol if you have kidney or liver problems. Don't take more than one product containing paracetamol at a time.

Aspirin (acetylsalicylic acid) This is effective against mild to moderate pain and it reduces fever. It works by blocking the production of inflammatory chemicals in the body through the inhibition of an enzyme known as cyclo-oxygenase-1 (COX-1). It's suitable for most types of arthritis, especially those associated with inflammation, but it's usually avoided in cases of gout because it can increase the blood level of uric acid to precipitate an attack in some people. Aspirin is best taken in soluble, effervescent, or enteric-coated form to minimize stomach irritation. It's not usually advised for children under the age of 16, for pregnant or breastfeeding women, or for people with a history of peptic ulcers, asthma, or a blood-clotting disorder. Check with a doctor before taking aspirin if you have gout, asthma, kidney or liver problems, or if you are on any other medication (drug interactions are common).

Benorilate This is a chemical cross between paracetamol and aspirin: 2 g benorilate contains just over 1 g of aspirin, and just under 1 g paracetamol. It's effective against mild to moderate pain.

Nonsteroidal anti-inflammatory drugs (NSAIDs)

In single or low doses, NSAIDs act as painkillers, with a similar effect as paracetamol on mild to moderate pain. They can also reduce fever. In regular or higher doses NSAIDs have an additional anti-inflammatory action to reduce redness, stiffness, and swelling. They are used in high doses to treat acute attacks of gout.

Although NSAIDs were widely prescribed to treat all types of arthritis, their use is now limited by their potential for side effects. These side effects range

Cartilage transplants

If you have osteoarthritis, cartilage cells can be harvested from one of your healthy joints, grown in the laboratory, and transplanted back into a joint whose cartilage is damaged. The chondrocytes (cartilage-making cells) then produce a healthy new joint lining, although it's not yet clear how long this new cartilage is likely to last.

from gastric irritation to worsening existing asthma in some people. NSAIDs have also been associated with kidney and cardiovascular problems. As a result, you shouldn't take NSAIDs (except under supervision) if you have a history of peptic ulcers or asthma, or you are pregnant or breastfeeding. Check with a pharmacist for interactions if you are taking other drugs.

Topical painkillers These are painkillers you can massage gently into the skin. Some topical painkillers, called rubefacients, contain substances that cause continuous, low-level stimulation of the skin, bringing increased blood flow, warmth, and redness. This helps to reduce the transmission of pain signals from the underlying joint. Rubefacients typically include substances such as menthol or methyl salicylate (oil of wintergreen), or capsaicin (from chili peppers).

Some NSAIDs are also available as topical creams or gels, and sink through the skin to the underlying joint to reduce pain and inflammation.

Transcutaneous electrical nerve stimulation (TENS)
This is a drug-free way to relieve pain. A typical TENS machine contains four pads that are stuck to your back, or around a painful joint. The device then generates small pulses of electric current that stimulate your

nerve endings. This sends pain-blocking signals to the brain and temporarily numbs surrounding tissues in a similar way to acupuncture.

Corticosteroids These are synthetic drug forms of the adrenal hormones that are involved in the body's response to stress. In nature, steroid hormones allow you to perform feats of endurance with little perception of pain. They have a powerful anti-inflammatory action to reduce pain and swelling. They can also damp down abnormal immune processes, such as those involved in rheumatoid arthritis.

You can take corticosteroid drugs orally or have them injected directly into a joint. The long-term use of oral corticosteroids is limited by their potential side effects, which include bone thinning, glucose intolerance, and weight gain. However, short, sharp oral courses (seven to 10 days) of a corticosteroid called prednisolone can provide considerable benefits with minimal risk of side effects. And some evidence suggests low-dose prednisolone (7.5 mg daily) can reduce the rate of joint destruction in early, moderate-to-severe rheumatoid arthritis if you take it for two to four years.

If you take oral corticosteroids for longer than three weeks, you are usually given a steroid treatment card that warns against stopping treatment suddenly—the dose should always be tapered off to allow recovery from any suppression of your adrenal glands.

Injections of corticosteroid drugs can reduce pain and inflammation, but repeated injections, especially into a weight-bearing joint, such as the knee, can lead to joint degeneration. Most doctors prefer not to inject a joint more than three times.

Opioid drugs If you have severe joint pain, you might be prescribed stronger morphine-related painkillers, such as fentanyl or buprenorphine. They usually come in the form of skin patches that slowly release the drug into your circulation. Opiates have a direct action on pain perception in the brain. Other opiate-related drugs include codeine and dihydrocodeine. They work well in combination with paracetamol for occasional use when pain flares up, but they cause constipation if you use them regularly. They can also be addictive.

Possible side effects of opiates include nausea, vomiting, constipation, drowsiness, headache, flashing, dizziness, and palpitations. Patches can cause redness, rash, or itching at the site of application.

Disease-modifying antirheumatic drugs (DMARDs)

DMARDs are a motley collection of unrelated drugs that interfere with different aspects of the immune response. They are prescribed as early as possible in autoimmune joint diseases, such as rheumatoid arthritis, psoriatic arthropathy, and ankylosing spondylitis, because they may reduce the progressive destruction of inflamed joints.

The action of DMARDs isn't completely understood, but we know they affect white-blood-cell function to damp down abnormal immune reactions. It can take several weeks for DMARDs to produce an effect.

Drugs in this group include gold salts (sodium aurothiomalate and auranofin), penicillamine, leflunomide, sulfasalazine (an antibiotic), some anti-rejection drugs used in tissue transplants (azathioprine and ciclosporin), some anticancer drugs (methotrexate and cyclophosphamide), and some antimalaria drugs (chloroquine and hydrochloroquine). The potential for side effects is high: you'll need regular checks to monitor your blood pressure, blood count, and liver and kidney function while taking DMARDs.

Biological Response Modifiers (BMRs)

If a DMARD doesn't work for someone with an autoimmune form of arthritis, doctors might recommend a BMR. These inhibit the production or action of cytokines (chemicals secreted by white blood cells during inflammation). BMRs are given by injection or by infusion. They can

. . . .

How opioid drugs relieve pain

Opioid drugs both reduce the transmission of pain signals and affect the way pain is perceived. Although pain can still be present, it no longer seems to matter.

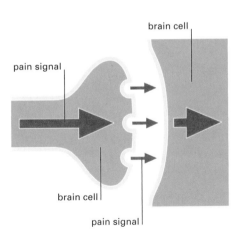

Before taking opioid drug

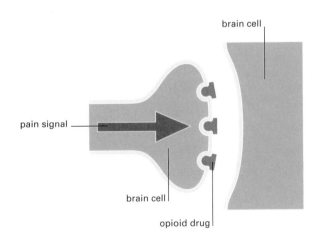

After taking opioid drug

Ninety percent of people undergoing joint replacement report rapid pain relief, improved mobility, and better quality of life.

relieve rheumatoid arthritis, psoriatic arthropathy, or ankylosing spondylitis in some people, but are stopped if there is not any improvement within three months.

Because BMRs reduce your immune response, they increase the risk of serious infections, such as tuberculosis, pneumonia, and septicemia. Other potential side effects include nausea, headache, abdominal pain, allergic reactions, blood disorders, and injection-site reactions. Because the potential for side effects is high, you usually have regular health checks while taking BMRs. You should tell your doctor if you are in contact with someone who has chickenpox or shingles.

Other drugs used to treat arthritis

If you have septic arthritis, you'll be treated with antimicrobial drugs, according to the bacteria, virus, or fungus that's responsible for your infection. The usual cause is a bacterium, which is treatable by antibiotics such as oxacillin, nafcillin, vancomycin, or cefotaxime. The septic joint is also drained. If your arthritis results from Lyme disease, tetracycline antibiotics can help.

A variety of medicines are used to treat gout (in addition to high doses of NSAIDs). Colchicine, a poison originally derived from the autumn crocus, reduces the pain and inflammation of gout, but is used only on a short-term basis, because it has arseniclike side effects such as vomiting and abdominal pain. It's often used to relieve gout symptoms as you begin longer-term treatment with allopurinol. This insures gout doesn't recur before allopurinol achieves its full effect. Allopurinol is used only after an acute attack has subsided as, paradoxically, it makes an acute attack worse. Side effects of allopurinol are rare, but can include rashes, allergic reactions, hepatitis, and kidney problems. Another drug, sulfinpyrazone, can treat gout, but a potential side effect is the production of uric-acid kidney stones.

Surgery

When pain and disability are severe enough to damage your quality of life, and drug treatment hasn't worked, your doctor might recommend surgery.

Synovectomy This is the removal of the inflamed, thickened synovial membrane that can overgrow and invade the joint in rheumatoid arthritis. This procedure can improve joint mobility and reduce pain and inflammation. Depending on how much excess membrane needs to be removed, this procedure can occur through a small incision; during joint keyhole surgery (arthroscopy); or during an open operation in which the whole joint is exposed. The procedure can provide relief for one or more years and postpone the need for joint replacement.

Osteotomy This involves the removal of a section of bone to realign a joint and correct deformity. It can improve pain and mobility in osteoarthritic joints, such as the knee; in vertebral joints stiffened by ankylosing spondylitis; and in joints, such as the hip, that are deformed by rheumatoid arthritis. It can take several months to recover from osteotomy, but the benefits usually last years. The procedure can make future joint replacement more difficult, because it alters your joint anatomy.

Arthrodesis This is the removal or fusion of a joint so your bones lock into place. The procedure stabilizes the joint and relieves pain in joints involving the vertebral column, thumb, and wrist. Hip, knee, and ankle joints can also be fused into a position that allows optimal function, so you can walk well, but with a limp. Weight-bearing joints are usually fused in cases where joint replacement is unsuitable; for example, because of osteoporosis or abnormal anatomy from a congenital dislocation of the hip or a deformed fracture.

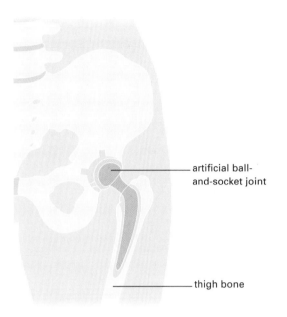

artificial ball-and-socket joint

thigh bone

Hip replacement
During hip replacement, part of your thigh bone is removed and replaced with a metal shaft and ball. The ball fits into a plastic socket that's inserted into your pelvis.

Arthroplasty This is the replacement of damaged parts of a joint with a new, artificial prosthesis. The joints most usually replaced include the ankle, finger, hip, knee, elbow, and shoulder. In most cases, the whole joint is replaced, with metal and plastic surfaces replacing all the bone and cartilage within a joint, while in others, just one part of the joint might need to be renewed, such as in hip resurfacing, where the ball-shaped head of the femur is preserved, reshaped, and capped with a metal prosthesis.

You are encouraged to use a new joint soon after arthroplasty, often the next day. Ninety percent of people undergoing joint replacement report rapid pain relief, improved mobility, and better quality of life.

The natural health approach

The natural health approach to treating arthritis involves a number of **complementary therapies** that you can use in conjunction with the treatment your doctor prescribes. These include aromatherapy, herbal medicine, naturopathy, hydrotherapy, homeopathy, and reflexology. I also take you through the principles of **manipulation therapies**, such as chiropractic and osteopathy, and explain how **Eastern approaches**, such as acupuncture, yoga, and qigong, can help alleviate joint pain. Magnets and copper are very popular in the treatment of arthritis and I explain how you can put these to practical use. **Tackling arthritis through the food you eat is important, too**—by following a diet that is rich in antioxidants, and by avoiding foods that may act as a trigger for your arthritis, you can reduce the level of inflammation in your joints. Simple measures such as **eating more fruit, vegetables, and oily fish** can go a long way to help. Some dietary supplements, such as glucosamine, are extremely beneficial. You may also find that **lifestyle changes** can provide symptom relief—I explain how you can start exercising in ways that won't hurt your joints, and how to reduce your weight if you need to—losing weight is a very effective way of relieving pressure on your joints.

complementary approaches to treatment

There are a number of therapies you can use to complement the orthodox treatment of arthritis. These include practitioner-led therapies, such as Reiki, osteopathy, and chiropractic, and approaches in which you will benefit from initial professional guidance, such as naturopathy and herbal medicine, before continuing by yourself at home. Several self-help therapies are, also beneficial, such as hydrotherapy, and magnetic and copper therapy.

Over the next few pages I explore the main complementary therapies used to treat all forms of arthritis. Some, such as aromatherapy, meditation, and yoga, work mainly through relaxation, which reduces strain on muscles, ligaments, and joints; while others, such as acupuncture, reflexology, and homeopathy, harness your body's own natural healing abilities to reduce pain. In contrast, herbal medicine uses plant extracts that have a physiological effect on the body, modifying its function in a similar way to some prescribed anti-inflammatory drugs.

In many cases, complementary therapies can improve your symptoms enough to reduce your need to take orthodox painkillers. This is important because some painkillers, such as nonsteroidal anti-inflammatory drugs (NSAIDs) are associated with a number of adverse side effects (see pages 19–20).

Check therapists' credentials

If you choose to visit a therapist, it's important to consult someone who has the appropriate credentials. Ask a potential therapist about his or her qualifications, and experience and successes in treating arthritis. Make sure the therapist is accredited with the appropriate umbrella organization; and check he or she carries indemnity insurance. Alternatively, look for a therapist via an umbrella organization—most will send you a list of their qualified practitioners. Many organizations also have a facility on their website to help you find a therapist in your area. Some useful contact details are provided in the resource section of this book (see pages 174–175).

Consulting a therapist

Having checked the qualifications of your chosen therapist (see box on the left), find out how long your course of treatment is likely to last, and how much it's likely to cost, before you commit yourself to an appointment.

Once you receive guidance from a therapist, you might find you need only one or two consultations before you can treat yourself at home. If you visit a homeopath or an aromatherapist, for example, you can simply carry on taking the remedies they prescribe for you or, in the case of aromatherapy, experiment with your own essential-oil blends. Other therapies, particularly those that rely on hands-on treatments, such as reflexology, massage, chiropractic, and osteopathy, require you to attend regular appointments so you continue to experience benefits.

aromatherapy

Aromatherapy is one of the most popular complementary therapies for arthritis. The aromatic essential oils produced by the leaves, stems, bark, flowers, roots, or seeds of many plants have a natural, painkilling action or a muscle-relaxant effect to reduce spasms. As essential oils are highly concentrated, you must first dilute them with a carrier oil, such as almond, avocado, calendula, grapeseed, jojoba, or wheatgerm oil, before putting them on your skin.

Useful essential oils

If you have osteoarthritis, any of the following essential oils might help: basil, black pepper, coriander, ginger, lemon, marjoram, peppermint, and thyme. If you have autoimmune arthritis (rheumatoid or psoriatic arthritis, for example), choose from any of these essential oils: benzoin, camomile (German and Roman), eucalyptus, peppermint, geranium, lavender, lemon, rosemary, and thyme.

The following blend is useful for all types of arthritis (and can also help to reduce depression): eight drops each of eucalyptus and lavender oil mixed with four drops each of marjoram, peppermint and rosemary oil. Mix this blend with 100 ml carrier oil (blended from 45 ml almond oil, 45 ml apricot oil, and 10 ml jojoba oil). A lavender and rosemary oil blend (diluted with a carrier oil) might also be helpful.

How to use essential oils

Essential oils can be inhaled from a tissue or diffused into the atmosphere using a candle-lit burner, but your joints will benefit most from the direct methods of application described below. If you apply heat to your joint (by using a hot compress or during a hot bath), it's important to move the joint as much as possible immediately afterward. This helps you derive maximum

Use essential oils with caution

- Don't take essential oils internally.
- Before using an essential oil blend, put a small amount on a patch of skin and leave it for at least an hour to check it doesn't cause an adverse reaction.
- Don't use essential oils if you have high blood pressure or epilepsy, or if you are pregnant (or likely to be), except under supervision.
- Don't use undiluted oils on your skin.
- Keep essential oils away from the eyes.
- Essential oils are flammable, so don't put them on an open flame.

benefits from the heat treatment, and it also prevents congestion, which can make joint stiffness worse.

Massage oil To make a massage oil, add one to three drops of your chosen essential-oil blend to 5 ml carrier oil. For a larger quantity add 30 to 40 drops to 100 ml carrier oil. Massage into painful joints.

Aromatherapy bath Add five drops of essential oil/s to 15 ml carrier oil and mix. Run your bath so it's comfortably hot, then add the oil mix. Close the bathroom door to keep in the vapors, and soak for 15 to 20 minutes, preferably in candlelight.

Hot compress Fill a medium-size bowl with comfortably hot water and add six drops of your chosen essential oil/s. Fold a piece of clean, cotton cloth and dip it into the bowl. Squeeze out some of the excess water, but not too much. Place the hot, wet cloth over the painful joint until it cools down to body temperature. Repeat this simple procedure two or three times.

herbal medicine

Herbalism is one of the most effective complementary therapies for treating arthritis. Herbalists use different parts of different plants, depending on which has the highest concentration of active ingredients.

Herbal treatments

Herbal treatments for arthritis are best prescribed by a medical herbalist, but you can also buy herbal products. Choose "standardized" products, which means the remedy contains a consistent amount of active ingredient so each dose provides the same pain-relieving or anti-inflammatory benefits.

Arnica (*Arnica montana*) Herbalists use this mountain flower to make a topical gel. Research shows it's as effective as ibuprofen gel for treating painful joints.
Typical use: apply it two to four times a day.

Bromelain This enzyme from pineapple stems has an anti-inflammatory action. It can significantly reduce acute knee pain, stiffness, and swelling associated with osteoarthritis and rheumatoid arthritis. It can also reduce pain and bruising after surgery (consult your surgeon if you'd like to try it). Avoid it if you are taking blood-thinning medication, such as aspirin or warfarin.
Typical dose: 250–500 mg three times a day. Select supplements with at least 2,000 milk-clotting units.

Devil's claw (*Harpagophytum procumbens*) This eases pain and is as effective as a nonsteroidal, anti-inflammatory drug (NSAID). Avoid it if you have peptic ulcers or indigestion.
Typical dose: 1–10 g daily (depending on concentration of extract—to provide around 50 mg harpagoside daily).

Frankincense (*Boswellia dalzielii*) This contains anti-inflammatory substances called boswellic acids, which are as effective at relieving pain as many NSAIDs.
Typical dose: 200–400 mg two or three times a day, standardized for at least 37.5 percent boswellic acids.

Ginger (*Zingiber officinale*) This relieves joint pain by suppressing the release of inflammatory chemicals. It has a cartilage-protecting action and eases the pain of knee osteoarthritis on standing and after walking.
Typical dose: powdered gingerroot standardized for 0.4 percent volatile oils; 250 mg two to four times daily.

Olive (*Olea europaea*) Olive leaf extracts contain anti-inflammatory antioxidants that can decrease pain in people with osteoarthritis, and reduce inflammation in those with rheumatoid arthritis.
Typical dose: 400 mg a day.

Rosehip (*Rosa canina*) The extracts can reduce the pain and stiffness associated with rheumatoid and osteoarthritis by more than 80 percent.
Typical dose: 2.5 g once or twice a day.

Turmeric (*Curcuma longa*) The active ingredient curcumin has a powerful anti-inflammatory action equivalent to that of some prescribed corticosteroids.
Typical dose: 500–1,200 mg daily, standardized to 95 percent curcuminoids.

White willow (*Salix alba*) The bark of the white willow contains salicylic acid, the parent compound from which aspirin is synthesized. Although slower acting, white willow offers similar pain relief to aspirin, but with less risk of stomach irritation. Avoid if you have peptic ulcers, asthma, or are sensitive to aspirin.
Typical dose: 150–300 mg every six hours.

naturopathy

Naturopathy employs a range of therapies that help you maintain a healthy balance between your body's biochemistry and structure, and your emotions. The theory that underpins naturopathy is that once your body and mind are in equilibrium, they become able to heal themselves. A naturopath uses a variety of complementary approaches, including nutritional medicine, herbal remedies, hydrotherapy, massage, homeopathy, reflexology, relaxation techniques, hypnotherapy, and yoga. Many naturopaths are also trained in osteopathy or chiropractic manipulation.

Healthy diet and lifestyle

The goal of naturopathy is to identify and treat the cause of a disease rather than to suppress the symptoms. In the case of arthritis, naturopaths believe an accumulation of toxic acids in the joints is responsible. They recommend you reduce your intake of highly refined, processed foods, saturated animal fats, sugar, and salt; eat more fruit, vegetables, and wholegrains; and drink sufficient water. Other advice might include avoiding certain foods, such as foods from the nightshade family (see page 51), red meat (see pages 51–52), or dairy products. You might be advised to follow an alkaline diet (see pages 52–53). A naturopath is also likely to recommend supplements, such as omega-3 fish oils, glucosamine, chondroitin, MSM, calcium, magnesium, copper, and the herbs ginger, Boswellia, and Devil's claw. You can use fresh ginger to make a healing tea.

As well as dietary treatment, a naturopath can offer hydrotherapy treatments, plus advice on getting plenty of sleep and regular exercise, and finding ways to relax. There's an emphasis in naturopathy on the importance of fresh air, sunshine, a clean environment, a stress-free lifestyle, and a positive mental attitude.

Bee venom therapy

Some naturopaths use bee venom to treat arthritis. Bee venom contains a mix of chemicals that, paradoxically, can relieve joint and muscle pain in arthritic and rheumatic conditions. The venom is harvested using a mild electrostimulant technique that doesn't harm the bees. Treatment is via either injections combined with local anesthetic, typically into acupuncture points, or a topical balm. The balm often contains other natural ingredients such as capsaicin (from chili peppers) and tea tree oil. When applied to a painful joint twice a day, the balm stimulates the release of cortisol—one of the body's most powerful, natural anti-inflammatory hormones—and has an analgesic, anti-inflammatory and immune-boosting effect. When given by injection, you will experience stinging, swelling, and aching for several hours. Avoid bee venom therapy if you're allergic to bee stings, or have health problems, such as high blood pressure.

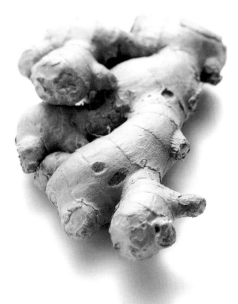

hydrotherapy

Hydrotherapy uses water as a healing substance, whether in the form of hot or cold liquid, steam, or ice. Temperature plays an important role in hydrotherapy, as both heat and cold have analgesic effects. Cold baths stimulate the metabolism and help reduce or prevent swelling and inflammation by constricting blood vessels. Warm water at body temperature is used to reduce sensory perception in floatation therapy; and hot water boosts circulation, helps muscles relax, eases aching joints, and reduces stiffness. Some treatments use hot and cold water alternately to reduce muscle spasm and boost production of the anti-inflammatory hormone cortisone.

Researchers have found that having a warm bath plus an ice massage can significantly raise pain thresholds in people with rheumatoid arthritis—the effect occurs immediately. They found that cryotherapy (application of ice) alone also has an immediate effect on pain threshold and lasts for 30 minutes. In people with osteoarthritis of the knee, having a 20-minute ice massage, five days a week for three weeks improves the strength of the quadriceps muscle by about 30 percent, and the range of knee flexion by eight percent. Another study showed that cold packs effectively reduce knee swelling.

Hydrotherapy techniques

Hydrotherapy uses a variety of different techniques, including bathing in mineral solutions, seaweed extracts (thalassotherapy), mud, peat, spa waters or sea water, and swimming in a pool. Therapists can also recommend a sitz bath (in which you immerse your buttocks, thighs, and lower back in water), saunas, steam rooms, whirlpools, hot tubs, high-pressure jets, hot compresses, wraps, ice packs, and aromatherapy baths. All can ease the pain of arthritis.

Exercising in water Hospital physiotherapy departments often offer exercise sessions in a warm swimming pool (typically at a temperature of 91.4–98.6°F). The warmth relaxes your muscles, and the buoyancy of the water reduces your body weight by 85 percent, which takes pressure off your joints making it easier to exercise. Moving your arms and legs against the water also offers enough resistance to help improve muscle strength. This kind of exercise is beneficial for people with all types of arthritis, but people with rheumatoid arthritis find it particularly beneficial. When 115 people with rheumatoid arthritis received either weekly 30-minute sessions of hydrotherapy or similar exercises on land, 87 percent of those treated with hydrotherapy reported they were "much better" or "very much better," compared with only 48 percent of those treated with land exercise.

Self-help hydrotherapy
You can recreate some of the effects of floatation therapy at home using mineral salts from the Dead Sea (available from some health-food stores and drug stores). Add a small envelope (9 ounces) Dead Sea salts to a warm bath and relax for 20 minutes (don't get the water in your eyes). Then wrap yourself in a warm towel and lie down in a warm room. Another useful hydrotherapy technique is to exercise your hands in a bowl of hot soapy water. Just open and close your hands and wriggle your fingers until they start to loosen up. Do this every morning to ease stiffness at the start of the day. Taking a hot bath or shower during the day can also ease pains and help maintain your mobility. If you find it difficult getting in and out of the bath, consider investing in grab rails, a bath lift, or a walk-in bath.

Hot and cold packs A therapist might recommend you use hot and cold gel-packs to ease joint pain and stiffness—you put the packs in either the microwave or the freezer. Some commercially available heat pads also contain magnets for additional benefits (see page 34). If you don't have a gel-pack, a bag of frozen peas can work as well, easily molding to the shape of an affected joint. My guidelines for when to use ice and when to use heat are as follows:

- If your joint is swollen and painful, use an ice pack.
- If your joint is stiff, but not swollen, use a heat pack.
- If you have an acute injury (one that happened within the last six weeks) use an ice pack.
- If in doubt, use ice first. If this isn't as effective as you would like, try a heat pack instead.

When using an ice pack, take care to avoid freezer burn. Instead of applying an ice pack directly to your skin, wrap it in a cloth and apply for up to 10 minutes at a time, then remove for a few minutes and re-apply.

Floatation therapy This involves lying in a lightproof, sound-insulated tank that contains a shallow, super-saturated solution of Epsom salts (magnesium sulfate). The minerals neutralize many of the effects of gravity, which helps you to relax completely—it's estimated that 90 percent of all brain activity is concerned with the effects of gravitational pull on the body, such as correcting posture and maintaining balance. The temperature of the floatation water is a constant 93.5°F (skin temperature).

You must be relatively mobile to have floatation therapy, because you need to climb safely in and out of the tank, which resembles an enclosed bath. Most people float naked, but you can wear a bathing suit if you prefer. Many large towns have a floatation center. For best results, try a course of five weekly floats.

How floatation therapy works

The tank screens out light and sound so your brain is cut off from virtually all external stimulation.

This induces a profoundly relaxed state in which you generate the special brainwaves—theta waves—associated with meditation, creative thought, and feelings of serenity. There is a significant increase in the secretion of endorphins, your brain's natural painkillers.

As well as relieving chronic pain, endorphins produce feelings of euphoria and improve the quality of your sleep.

The benefits last for up to three weeks. (In addition to easing arthritis symptoms, floatation therapy can lower high blood pressure.)

homeopathy

Homeopathy is based on the concept that like cures like—tiny amounts of a potential toxin can treat symptoms similar to those it would produce if used at full strength. Clinical trials show that homeopathy is significantly better than a placebo at treating arthritis.

Visiting a homeopath

A homeopath prescribes treatments according to your symptoms, personality, lifestyle, likes and dislikes, as well as your constitutional type. He or she will usually prescribe a 6c or 12c potency at first, followed by a higher potency (30c) if you experience partial symptom relief combined with a return of symptoms when you stop taking the remedy.

Take homeopathic remedies on their own without eating or drinking for at least 30 minutes before or afterward. If your symptoms worsen initially, persevere with treatment—it's a sign that a remedy is working. If there's no improvement after taking a remedy for the allotted time, consult your homeopath.

Homeopathic remedies for arthritis

These homeopathic remedies are often prescribed for people with arthritis, but a homeopath may prescribe others depending on your symptoms and your constitutional type.

remedy	prepared from	used to treat
Arnica	Leopard's bane/sneezewort	Arthritis in a joint previously damaged by trauma.
Apis	Honey bee	Hot, swollen, painful, stiff joints, especially the fingers and ankles.
Belladonna	Deadly nightshade	Septic arthritis with a hot, red, tender joint, plus fever.
Calcarea phosphorica	Calcium phosphate	Weakness and pain in the hips.
Colchicum	Meadow saffron	Gout with a red, hot, swollen, excruciatingly painful joint.
Kali iodatum	Potassium iodide	Swollen, painful knee joints, with symptoms worse at night and in damp weather.
Ledum	Wild rosemary/marsh tea	Arthritis that starts in the lower limbs and moves to joints in the upper body.
Lycopodium	Club moss	Recurrent attacks of gout in someone with arthritis in other joints, and frequent cramps.
Rhus toxicodendron	Poison ivy	Swollen, stiff joints that are initially painful then eased by movement.
Sabina	Juniper	Arthritis with red, shiny, swollen joints.
Urtica	Stinging nettle	Gout with stinging pains and itchiness.

copper therapy

When you wear copper jewelry, trace amounts of copper are absorbed through your skin. Many people find this is effective at easing their joint symptoms. It still isn't known exactly how copper exerts its therapeutic effect, but it's known that copper is involved in the synthesis of collagen—a major structural protein in bones and joints—and it's thought a lack of copper contributes to the development of inflammatory diseases. As well as being important for joint health, copper can have a direct analgesic effect.

How to use copper

Although you can get copper from your diet, the amounts present in food are tiny and most doesn't get absorbed. Foods with the highest copper concentrations include kidney, shellfish, nuts, seeds, legumes and wholegrains, and vegetables that have been grown in copper-rich soil. It's thought average copper intakes are about 1.6 mg a day, but, of this, 70 percent isn't absorbed by the gut because copper becomes bound to other bowel contents, such as sugars, sweeteners, and refined flour.

Copper is much more readily absorbed through the skin. Wearing copper products, however, doesn't help everyone with arthritis. The effectiveness of a copper product is thought to depend on the level of copper already present in your body. If you are copper-deficient, you might benefit; but if your levels are already adequate, copper products might not help.

For copper to work properly, you need to have adequate levels of zinc in your body. The ideal dietary ratio of copper to zinc is one to 10. I recommend you obtain at least 15 mg of zinc a day from your diet or that you take zinc supplements. Zinc is found in seafood, particularly oysters. Even if you don't use copper products, zinc is a useful mineral for people with rheumatoid arthritis (see page 61).

Copper jewelry When you wear copper jewelry, such as bracelets or rings, copper is absorbed through your skin at an estimated rate of 100–150 mg copper a year. In one study of more than 300 people with a variety of types of arthritis, copper bracelets worn on the wrists and ankles were analyzed to see how much copper they lost over a period of 50 days. Results showed that they lost between 80 and 90 mg. Participants in the study reported positive benefits as a result of wearing the bracelets. Interestingly, some other participants in the study, who wore a placebo bracelet (having previously worn an authentic copper one), experienced a significant deterioration in their arthritis symptoms. In another trial involving 240 people with rheumatoid arthritis, those wearing copper bracelets experienced a statistically significant reduction in their arthritis symptoms when compared with participants wearing a placebo bracelet.

Expect a slight green discoloration of your skin when you wear copper jewelry, which is caused by the interaction of copper and sweat.

Copper shoe inserts

Try wearing shoe inserts made from copper. The inserts, developed by a podiatrist, are called "Copper Heelers" (see page 159) and they fit easily into your shoes. It's thought acid sweat from your feet hastens the absorption of copper through your soles. Anecdotal evidence suggests that the product significantly reduces joint pain.

magnetic therapy

Applying a magnet to an arthritic joint can help in a number of ways. First, it encourages small blood vessels to dilate and causes iron-containing red blood cells to line up in the same direction so they pass through blood capillaries more easily. This increases blood flow to the affected joint.

Second, magnetized red blood cells are able to carry oxygen more efficiently, so the joint receives more oxygen and nutrients, and toxins are removed more easily. Finally, magnets help to damp down inflammation and pain, and they stimulate the production of the body's natural painkillers (endorphins). Research shows that exposure to a static magnet can increase endorphin levels by 25 percent within one hour and by 45 percent within two hours.

A study in Japan involving 121 patients with severe, chronic shoulder pain revealed that 82 percent of those using high-strength magnets showed significant improvement within four days. In those treated with low-strength magnets, there was only a 37-percent improvement rate.

Using magnets therapeutically

Therapeutic magnets are widely used to alleviate the pain of arthritis and other inflammatory conditions. They often take the form of jewelry or shoe in-soles. You can also buy magnetic wraps to wrap around joints, such as the knee, ankle, or elbow. The wraps are secured with Velcro and they don't restrict your movement. As well as providing magnetic therapy, they also give support to a painful joint. Adhesive magnetic patches are available, too. You can use patches in the following ways:

- Stick them over acupuncture points near the site of pain. Consult an acupuncturist for advice.
- Stick the patches directly on any areas of tenderness.
- Stick several patches on the skin so they surround the painful joint.

When buying a magnet, choose one that's strong enough to have a therapeutic effect. The strength of a magnetic field is measured in units known as teslas or gauss. One tesla is equivalent to 10,000 gauss. Magnets that are used for healing have field strengths that range from 200–2000 gauss (20 to 200 milliteslas). For optimum effect, I suggest you select a therapeutic magnet with a field strength of at least 500 gauss.

When to avoid magnetic therapy

Keep magnets away from computer disks and other magnetic media. Do not use magnets:

- If you have an infection.
- If you have recently had chicken pox.
- On open wounds, except under medical supervision.
- If you have hemophilia.
- If you have a heart pacemaker.
- If you are undergoing dialysis.
- If you are using an insulin pump or drug patch. (Use magnets only under medical supervision.)
- If you have a surgically implanted metal screw in your body.
- If you are pregnant or trying to conceive.

massage

As well as encouraging general relaxation, massage eases muscle tension and stimulates the release of endorphins—the body's natural painkillers. People with all forms of arthritis can benefit from regular massage.

Visiting a massage therapist

During a massage, you usually lie on a massage table with a hole over which you rest your head. Alternatively, you can sit, leaning forward in a massage chair, or lie on a pad on the floor. The part of the body to be massaged is usually uncovered, but you can wear clothes during some techniques, such as acupressure, shiatsu, tui na, and Thai massage.

Types of massage

A massage therapist uses a variety of strokes to stimulate the soft tissues, such as rubbing, drumming, kneading, wringing, friction, and applying deep pressure. More than 100 different types of massage are recognized. Any of the following types might help relieve your symptoms. Be sure to tell your massage therapist you have arthritis, prior to a massage.

Swedish massage A therapist uses massage oil and lotion. Strokes are long, smooth, and gentle.

Aromatherapy massage This combines Swedish massage with essential oils selected for your particular joint symptoms (see page 27).

Ayurvedic massage One or more therapists rub warm, herb-infused medicinal oil into every part of your body, including your scalp.

.

Bowen technique This uses rolling movements over muscles, ligaments, tendons, and joints.

Deep tissue massage This focuses on a specific joint, muscle, or muscle group. Therapists use their fingers, knuckles, elbows, and thumbs, as well as the heel of the hand and even the foot to massage deeper into a problem area, ease muscle spasm, and improve movement and mobility.

Hot stone massage Therapists warm smooth stones, such as basalt or marble, in water, then coat them in oil and use them to massage and relax your muscles.

Myofascial release This stretches the tissue layer (fascia) that binds muscles together, allowing them to move more freely.

Shiatsu This is a Japanese form of massage in which practitioners use their fingers and thumbs to massage and stimulate acupressure points on the skin. Each point is held for a few seconds.

Thai massage More energetic than other forms, Thai massage involves stretching your body into a series of yogalike postures. The practitioner uses their hands, forearms, and feet to apply firm, rhythmic pressure, including pulling fingers, toes, and ears.

Tui na This is a form of Chinese massage in which muscles are pushed, pulled, stretched, and kneaded.

Rolfing Also known as structural integration, this combines massage with deep pressure and postural adjustments in which the therapist slowly stretches and repositions your body's supportive soft tissues.

Hellerwork This is a modern adaptation of Rolfing, in which massage and postural adjustments are combined with exploration of the emotions triggered by the release of tension.

osteopathy

Osteopathy involves gentle manipulation of the muscles, ligaments, and joints to help relax muscles, correct poor alignment, and reduce pain.

Osteopathy can help to treat all types of arthritis, and is effective at reducing pain, especially in the neck, lower back, and hip. It can also reduce early morning stiffness and joint swelling, and improve joint movement, and mobility. In fact, research suggests spinal manipulation is more effective than either painkillers or exercise for treating back pain, with most people reporting striking benefits. A study published in the *New England Journal of Medicine*, in 1999, concluded osteopathic manipulation is as effective as standard medical care with painkillers, application of heat and cold, and the use of a TENS machine (see page 20). On average, people receiving osteopathy were found to have achieved a 30-percent reduction in the level of their pain. Half as many people with arthritis who received osteopathic treatment needed NSAID analgesics compared with those on standard care (24 percent versus 54 percent).

Visiting an osteopath

An osteopath will ask questions about your medical history, your general health, and the specific problems you're experiencing at the moment. He or she will then assess the range of movement in your joints, and palpate (feel) parts of your body to detect areas of weakness, misalignment, and excessive strain. The osteopath will also check your posture for symmetry and alignment of the pelvis, and compare the length of your legs. He or she will gently tap on muscle tendons at your knees, ankles, elbows, and/or wrists to test your nerve reflexes. If necessary, you may have additional investigations, such as x-rays or blood tests.

Having got a full picture of your joint health, an osteopath will tailor a treatment plan to your needs. Osteopathic treatment involves manual manipulations that include gentle massage to relax tension, mobilization of stiff joints by stretching them rhythmically within their normal range of movement, and swift, high-velocity thrusts to correct poor bone alignments. Spinal manipulation can also sometimes involve using your limbs to make levered thrusts. An osteopath might also give you advice on posture and how to reduce strain when lifting. He or she might recommend wearing flat shoes and using ergonomic aids when sitting and working at a desk and computer.

Cranial osteopathy

This branch of osteopathy evolved from the understanding that the fused joints of the skull retain slight flexibility, so the head becomes slightly wider from side to side, and slightly shorter from front to back, when breathing in. Cranial osteopaths believe this happens to accommodate natural movements within the cerebrospinal fluid (CSF) that bathes and nourishes the brain and spinal cord, which is said to pulsate at six to 15 times per minute. Practitioners sense this pulsation (known as the cranial rhythmic impulse) with their hands and "listen" to the inner movements and tensions inside the patient. They use their highly trained sense of touch to identify disturbances in the joints of the skull, which are then manipulated using gentle but specific adjustments to improve the circulation of CSF, blood and lymph in the head. The technique is gentle enough to use on newborn babies, and can help a wide range of conditions, including back and neck pain, especially for severe problems where a doctor has advised against direct spinal manipulation.

chiropractic

Chiropractors specialize in the prevention, diagnosis, and treatment of mechanical disorders of the muscles and joints, and their adverse effects on the nervous system. They mainly focus on misalignments of the spinal vertebrae, known as subluxations, which are common in people with arthritis. These misalignments can pinch or stretch tiny nerves to cause pain and reduce mobility. Chiropractors use their hands to manipulate the spinal column and the joints in which movement is restricted.

Research has shown that combining chiropractic spinal manipulation with the application of moist heat (see page 31) is more effective in treating low-back pain caused by osteoarthritis than using heat alone. Chiropractic manipulation has also been shown to reduce pain in ankylosing spondylitis (see page 13), even where the sacroiliac joints and lumbar and cervical vertebrae are fused.

Visiting a chiropractor

A chiropractor asks questions about your medical history, lifestyle, diet, exercise patterns, work, current symptoms, and the type of bed you sleep on. He or she will observe your posture when you stand and walk, and will ask how you sit at a desk. During the examination you will be asked to variously stand, or sit, or lie on a chiropractic couch, and you will be maneuvered into a number of positions to assess your mobility and flexibility. This process, known as "motion palpation," helps the chiropractor assess which joints are moving freely, and which are stiff or locked. Motion palpation can identify the exact source of any pain that is troubling you. Irritation of a nerve in one area can sometimes lead to symptoms of discomfort in other parts of the body (known as referred pain), so manipulation might not be carried out at the site of

Craniosacral therapy
This involves the gentle manipulation of both the skull and the base of the spine. Craniosacral therapists believe the cranial rhythmic impulse (see box on page 36) affects every cell in the body. By gently manipulating and pressing on the head and sacrum, the therapist helps to achieve an even flow of the cranial rhythmic impulse, and facilitates the release of inner tensions over a wide area. Craniosacral therapy is used by many chiropractors—and osteopaths—to improve problems such as back and neck pain, headache, insomnia and stress.

your pain. Tingling in the fingers, for example, often results from misalignment (subluxation) of neck bones. A chiropractor might also use other diagnostic tests, such as x-rays, blood and urine tests, and MRI scans.

Your treatment will consist of rapid, direct, yet gentle, thrusts to correct vertebral subluxations. This helps bones to move into their correct positions, often with a click. This re-aligns muscles, tendons, ligaments, and joints to help relieve pain and tension. Sometimes, a rubber-tipped instrument known as an "activator" is used to gently manipulate the vertebrae, using small, precise, measured thrusts. Chiropractic also includes stretching and massage, if appropriate.

McTimoney chiropractic is similar to standard chiropractic in that it focuses on the spine and nervous system, but it also considers joints in other parts of the body. During a session, a McTimoney chiropractor will use his or her hands to check and adjust the spine, pelvis, chest, limbs, and skull. He or she will use a number of light, swift hand movements that are unique to McTimoney chiropractic, including gentle fingertip manipulation to realign joints.

reflexology

Reflexology is an ancient technique at least 5,000 years old, and is based on similar principles to acupressure. It involves the stimulation and massage of points, known as reflexes, on the feet and hands. Each reflex corresponds to a specific part of the body, in such a way that forms a map of the body on the hands and feet. Look at the illustrations of the hands (below) to see where specific areas are represented. Areas on your palms and the soles of your feet, for example, relate to your shoulders, sciatic nerves, and spine, while reflexes on the backs of your hands and the tops of your feet relate to your hips, knees, elbows, and sacroiliac joints. Reflexology can help to reduce

inflammation, relieve the symptoms of stress, and improve joint mobility and general well-being.

Visiting a reflexologist

During a reflexology session, a therapist massages all areas of your feet and/or hands using firm thumb and finger pressure. The therapist will then treat specific problems such as arthritis by applying pressure and

Reflexology hand maps

These maps show where specific areas of the body are represented on the fronts and backs of both hands. Massaging the areas that correspond to painful joints can help to relieve arthritis symptoms.

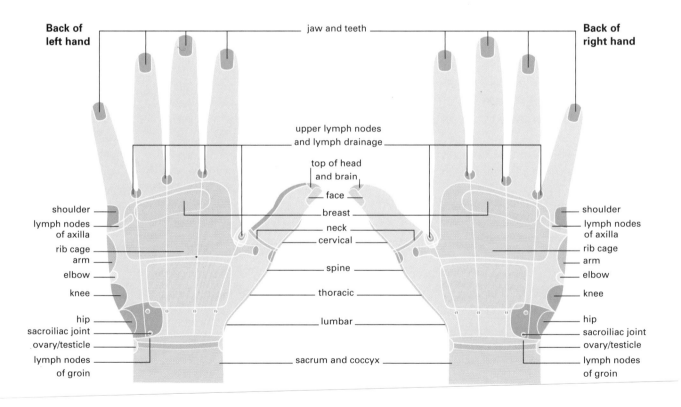

Back of left hand — jaw and teeth — **Back of right hand**

upper lymph nodes and lymph drainage
top of head and brain
face
shoulder — breast — shoulder
lymph nodes of axilla — neck — lymph nodes of axilla
rib cage — cervical — rib cage
arm — arm
elbow — spine — elbow
knee — thoracic — knee
hip — hip
sacroiliac joint — lumbar — sacroiliac joint
ovary/testicle — ovary/testicle
lymph nodes of groin — sacrum and coccyx — lymph nodes of groin

massaging the reflex points that correspond to the affected area. This stimulates nerve endings that pass from the hands or feet to the brain and out to the related part of the body, helping to reduce symptoms such as pain, swelling, and stiffness. The therapist might also massage reflexes corresponding to your adrenal glands to stimulate production of the anti-inflammatory hormone cortisone.

Full treatment usually lasts 45 to 60 minutes and at the end of each session you will feel warm, contented, and relaxed. For optimum benefit, have one session a week for two months, then decide whether you find the treatment helps your arthritis. I have included details of reflexology organizations at the end of this book (see page 175).

Self-help reflexology

You can help to ease your arthritis symptoms by gently massaging the knee, hip, and spinal reflexes on your hands. Your spinal reflexes run along the sides of your thumbs, with the cervical area starting level with the bottom of your nails, followed by the thoracic spine, then the lumbar region in the curve where your hands and wrists meet, then the sacrum and coccyx at the sides of your wrists. Feel along these areas and stop on any that are tender. Press the reflexes, gradually pushing harder (up to the limit of comfort). Maintain the pressure for at least 20 seconds, then press and release in quick pulses of one or two seconds. Do this twice a day, morning and evening.

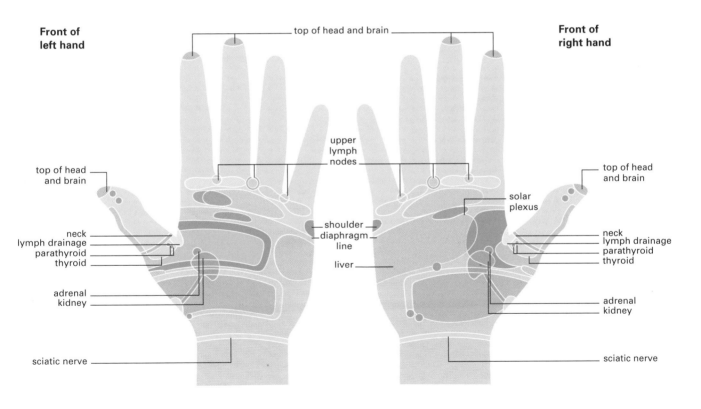

Front of left hand

Front of right hand

top of head and brain

top of head and brain

upper lymph nodes

top of head and brain

solar plexus

neck
lymph drainage
parathyroid
thyroid

shoulder
diaphragm line

neck
lymph drainage
parathyroid
thyroid

liver

adrenal
kidney

adrenal
kidney

sciatic nerve

sciatic nerve

yoga

Yoga, the ancient Eastern practice of movement, breathing, and meditation, is beneficial for arthritis because it improves muscle strength, suppleness, and range of movement. It also helps you to relax and manage pain. As well as the physical benefits, people who practice yoga regularly tend to enjoy feelings of emotional well-being and positivity, which can help you cope with the challenge of living with arthritis.

Starting yoga

Yoga is best practiced daily, but practicing a few times a week for 30 to 60 minutes per session will also be beneficial. Join a beginner's class and tell the yoga teacher you have arthritis. Once you've learned the basic postures and breathing techniques from a teacher, yoga is an excellent self-help therapy you can continue at home. Gradually build up your practice time over a period of weeks and months.

Don't push yourself beyond your limits in yoga. Learn to recognize the difference between the mild discomfort of stretching a muscle and the "bad" pain that comes from putting undue pressure on a joint.

Yoga is widely taught in the West—you'll find classes at gyms and leisure centers, complementary health centers, and dedicated yoga centers.

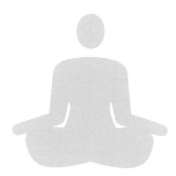

Types of yoga

There are many types of yoga, ranging from the strenuous (ashtanga yoga) to the gentle (viniyoga). I suggest you try any of following three types, which are the most suitable for people with arthritis.

Hatha yoga This is the most popular form of yoga in the West. It involves a series of simple poses that flow comfortably from one to another at your own pace. Hatha yoga can improve hand-grip strength, reduce joint tenderness ,and improve the range of finger movement in people with either rheumatoid arthritis or osteoarthritis of the hands. Even people with severe rheumatoid arthritis can benefit. Research shows that twice-weekly, hour-long hatha yoga sessions can ease chronic low-back pain and improve balance and flexibility, with the benefits lasting for several months.

Iyengar yoga This is a form of hatha yoga that's ideal if you have reduced flexibility. It employs items like chairs, blocks, and pillows to provide stability between your body and the floor if you're unable to bend fully into the postures. It's sometimes described as "meditation in action," because it focuses on symmetry, alignment, and meditation, with postures being held for longer periods than in most other forms of yoga. Research indicates that performing Iyengar yoga postures for 90 minutes once a week for eight weeks can reduce pain and stiffness and improve joint function in people with osteoarthritis of the knee. Lyengar yoga can also alleviate chronic low-back pain, reducing disability and use of pain medication.

Viniyoga This is also good for people with arthritis, because its slow, gentle movements don't stress the joints. Viniyoga uses breath awareness, relaxation, meditation, and guided imagery to reduce pain.

qigong

Qigong (pronounced "chee gong") is a traditional Chinese healing art that's sometimes referred to as "Chinese yoga" or "acupuncture without needles." It involves the use of gentle movements, stretches, guided imagery, and meditation to help you relax and breathe in a way that heals and nourishes the body. The basic postures of qigong are easy to learn and can be performed in any order. Qigong helps to strengthen your muscles and make you more supple. It also promotes feelings of lightness and calm that can help to improve your pain thresholds and help you live with arthritis on a day-to-day level.

Qigong is part of Traditional Chinese Medicine (TCM), which is based upon the belief life-force energy, or qi, circulates throughout the body in channels known as meridians (see the illustrations on page 43). Strengthening or balancing the flow of qi by practicing qigong (or by having acupressure or acupuncture) improves your health and reduces your susceptibility to disease. In China, qigong is widely used to treat arthritis, which is believed to result from the body being invaded by a type of qi called "wind-cold-damp qi," which causes a qi blockage in certain joints. Treatment, therefore, involves eradicating the wind-cold-damp qi, eliminating the qi blockage in the affected joint, and introducing healthy and balanced qi into the area.

Research shows that practicing the standing postures of qigong alleviates the symptoms of chronic rheumatoid arthritis. In one trial, significantly more people reported an improvement in their symptoms from practicing qigong than did those from a group treated with indomethacin (a strong nonsteroidal anti-inflammatory drug). Qigong can also help people with osteoarthritis of the hands, knee, or hip, and with spondylitis, and nonspecific muscle and joint pains.

Qigong walking

Particularly beneficial for arthritis, qigong walking uses more muscles than conventional walking. It encourages you to walk purposefully and slowly, and to move your arms as well as your legs in a smooth, relaxed rhythm. To practice qigong walking, bend your right arm and bring your right hand up to chest level (palm facing down, fingers naturally coiled in) as your left leg moves forward. Then swing your right arm down and back as you bring your left hand up and your right leg forward. Alternatively, try swaying your arms from one side of your body to the other in coordination with your step. As you step forward with your left foot, sway both arms to your left. As you step your right foot forward, sway both arms to your right. Once you've got the hang of the arm movements, focus on making your foot movements precise. Touch the ground with your heel first—toes pointing up—then roll your foot down. Breathing is important, too. Take in two small breaths as you step forward with your left foot, and breathe out in a single exhalation as you step forward with your right foot. After 20 minutes of walking, reverse this so you take two small inhalations as you step forward with your right foot and you exhale once as you step forward with your left foot. Do this for another 20 minutes.

Starting qigong

You can go to classes to learn qigong or you can also learn postures and techniques from books and videos. If you can't find a dedicated qigong class, look for a tai chi class—qigong postures often form part of the class. Alternatively, a tai chi teacher might be able to give you private qigong lessons. Try to practice qigong everyday to benefit from its therapeutic effects.

acupuncture

Acupuncture is based on the belief we all possess a vibrant life-energy, known as qi or chi (pronounced "chee") in China, and ki in Japan. Qi flows through the body along special channels called meridians and becomes concentrated at certain points, called acupoints, where it can enter or leave the body. There are 12 main meridians and eight meridians that have a controlling function, making 20 in all. Traditionally, 365 acupoints were identified on these meridians, but many more have now been discovered and about 2,000 acupoints are illustrated on modern acupuncture charts. During acupuncture, a therapist stimulates or suppresses the flow of qi by inserting needles into your skin.

Acupuncture is among the most widely used complementary therapies for treating arthritis. In the West, an estimated one in two of all consultations with an acupuncturist are for arthritic conditions.

Self-help acupressure

To help reduce joint pains in your hips and lower limbs, locate an area on the base of your palm that is about a thumb's width above the wrist crease. Press either side of the midline in this area of the palm and find the point that is most tender. Press this area with the thumb of your opposite hand. Start by pressing lightly, and gradually increase the pressure as much as you can tolerate. Then release the pressure gradually and build it up again to stimulate the area. Continue pressing for about one minute, while breathing slowly and deeply. If your joint pains are worse on the left side of your body, stimulate the point on your right hand for relief, and vice versa. Do this twice a day, morning and evening.

Acupuncture is especially useful in the early stages of arthritis before degenerative changes cause severe pain and restricted movement.

A study published in the medical journal *Rheumatology* showed acupuncture produced a significant reduction in pain from osteoarthritis of the hip or knee after an average of eight treatments over a six-month period. Other studies show acupuncture can relieve chronic low-back pain and neck and shoulder pain, and it's at least as effective as treatment with nonsteroidal anti-inflammatory drugs or physiotherapy.

Acupressure works on the same principles as acupuncture, but instead of inserting needles, you stimulate acupoints using firm thumb pressure or fingertip massage. You can perform acupressure on yourself (see box).

How acupuncture works

Acupuncture is believed to work by blocking the transmission of pain signals along nerve fibers, and by stimulating the release of the brain's own painkillers, called endorphins, which are related to morphine. It can also work by having an impact on part of the brain known as the limbic system, which is involved in decisions about whether or not a sensation is perceived as painful.

Visiting an acupuncturist

An initial consultation with an acupuncturist usually lasts from 45 to 60 minutes, with follow-up appointments lasting about 30 minutes. The practitioner will ask a number of questions about your symptoms, lifestyle, bodily functions, and your emotional and physical health. He or she will examine your tongue and check various pulses in your wrists. During treatment the practitioner inserts fine, sterile, disposable needles a few millimetres into your skin at selected acupoints. Needles are usually left in place for 10 to 30 minutes and might be occasionally flicked or rotated to stimulate qi and draw or disperse energy from the point. They are sometimes stimulated with electricity (a technique known as electroacupuncture) or by burning a small cone of strong-smelling, dried Chinese herb (usually wild mugwort) near to the acupoint to warm the skin. This is known as moxibustion and is believed to stimulate weak qi in areas that are cold or painful. Acupuncturists also stimulate acupoints using laser light from a pen-device.

For a complex, long-standing problem such as arthritis, you will benefit from having at least one or two treatments per week for two months. Ideally, treatment is given every other day, or even daily for acute arthritis. Most people notice an immediate benefit after just one or two treatments, while others may need up to four to six treatments. Information on how to find a practitioner is included at the end of this book.

. . . .

The meridians

Meridians are energy-conducting channels that run along the length of your body. An acupuncturist inserts needles into selected acupoints that lie along these channels. This heals the body by stimulating or suppressing the flow of qi.

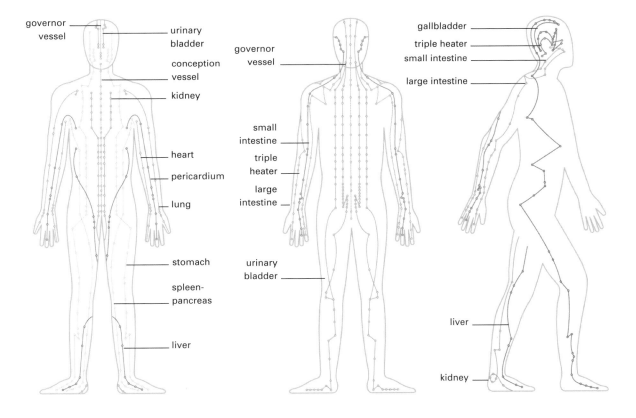

governor vessel
urinary bladder
conception vessel
kidney
heart
pericardium
lung
stomach
spleen-pancreas
liver

governor vessel
small intestine
triple heater
large intestine
urinary bladder

gallbladder
triple heater
small intestine
large intestine
liver
kidney

reiki

Reiki is a Japanese word meaning "universal life energy." It's a form of spiritual healing that has its roots in ancient Tibetan Buddhism and represents a simple, yet powerful way to promote emotional and physical harmony. A Reiki practitioner places their hands in a series of positions over or on your body, through which they channel and transmit the universal life energy ki. This energy is thought to help your body recover its normal state of physical and emotional wellness.

A number of studies suggest therapeutic touch therapies, such as Reiki, can help to reduce chronic pain and stress and improve well-being and energy levels. In one study of 82 people with osteoarthritis, pain intensity and distress were significantly reduced during the six-week period in which they received weekly Reiki sessions, compared with a similar period in which they practiced progressive muscle relaxation.

Visiting a Reiki practitioner

A typical treatment session takes 60 to 90 minutes, and involves the practitioner holding his or her hands over or on your fully clothed body in 12 basic positions: four on your head, four on the front of your body, and four on your back. The practitioner holds each position for around five minutes to balance your chakras (energy centers). There are seven chakras altogether, each of which is associated with a particular color (see the illustration on the right).

During a healing session, your body absorbs only as much Reiki energy as it needs. You might experience the flow of energy as a mild tingling or sense of warmth or coolness. Most people experience a deep sense of relaxation, peace, and well-being after treatment with Reiki. The benefits are increased by resting afterward and drinking plenty of water.

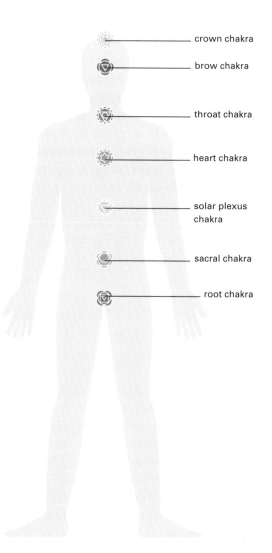

crown chakra

brow chakra

throat chakra

heart chakra

solar plexus chakra

sacral chakra

root chakra

The chakras

Life-force energy flows in to and out of the body via the chakras. When its flow is impeded, you become ill. The aim of Reiki is to restore the flow of energy in the chakras, bringing you health, and emotional and physical well-being. There are seven chakras and they lie along a line that runs from the perineum to the crown of your head.

the natural health approach

meditation

Meditation is a technique that involves focusing the mind to achieve a state of peaceful relaxation and heightened awareness. This helps you to cope better with the pain of arthritis, partly because your pain perception is reduced when you're in a meditative state, and partly because meditation improves your overall mood and sense of well-being.

Starting meditation

You can go to classes to learn meditation, you can learn one-to-one from a teacher, or you can simply start by yourself at home. Many yoga classes include a dedicated time for meditation. Ideally, you should meditate for 15 to 30 minutes for at least five days a week, and preferably every day.

Types of meditation

There are many different types of meditation—some derive from spiritual or religious backgrounds; some from secular backgrounds. These are some of the most common types in the West:

Mindfulness meditation This is one of the most popular forms of meditation, encouraging you to focus on the present moment. You pay close attention to everyday activities, such as preparing food or walking, and you concentrate your awareness on the sensations, textures, colors, smells, and sounds around you. Simply focusing on your breathing is also a form of mindfulness meditation. Being immersed in the moment prevents negative and stressful thoughts.

Moving meditation This is good if you have arthritis because it involves quieting your mind through gentle movements, such as walking along a set path, or rocking or swaying to and fro. These movements are designed to keep your body engaged while your mind becomes quiet. Qigong walking is an example of moving meditation (see the box on page 41).

Transcendental meditation This structured form of meditation, developed by Maharishi Mahesh Yogi in the 1950s, is practiced for 20 minutes twice a day. Transcendental meditation (TM) uses the silent repetition of Sanskrit mantras (short words or phrases) to still your thoughts and body so you achieve a state of restful alertness.

Relaxation response meditation This is a Westernized form of meditation that uses the principles of TM without the Eastern spiritual context. Instead of Sanskrit mantras, you silently chant words that are rooted in your own belief system. For example, relaxation exercises are combined with words such as "calm" or "peace."

Chakra meditation

Chakras are worked upon in a range of complementary therapies, from yoga and Reiki to meditation. To meditate upon the chakras sit comfortably with your eyes closed and then spend two minutes concentrating on each chakra, visualizing the color with which it is associated. Start by focusing on the root chakra (red) at the base of your spine, and imagine pulling energy up in a straight line through the sacral chakra (orange), solar plexus chakra (yellow), heart chakra (green), throat chakra (sky blue) to the brow chakra (violet). Now focus on drawing energy up toward the crown chakra (white) at the very top of your head. Finally, imagine energy flowing out of the top of your head, like a fountain, to envelop your body in a pain-relieving, healing white light.

nutritional approaches to treatment

Research shows a definite link between the food you eat and the severity of your arthritis symptoms. Here I explain some important dietary measures that can improve your joint health. See Part Three for practical ways to implement these.

Fruit and vegetables—eat at least five servings a day

Like your heart, your joints thrive best on plenty of fresh fruit and vegetables. Try to eat at least five (and preferably eight or more) servings a day. Fruit and vegetables provide an array of antioxidants that reduce the rate at which cartilage breaks down, helping to slow the progression of osteoarthritis. Antioxidants can also reduce inflammation and are beneficial for people with rheumatoid arthritis, psoriatic arthritis, ankylosing spondylitis, or gout. My full-strength program in the next section features a diet with the highest possible amount of antioxidants. (See also pages 47–49.)

Eat plenty of oily fish

Oily fish are a rich source of omega-3 essential fatty acids that oil the joints and damp down inflammation. Research shows that omega-3s can reduce the long-term need for painkillers in those with joint problems. Eat oily fish, such as salmon, sardines, herring, and mackerel, two to four times a week. You can also take an omega-3 fish-oil supplement (see page 61).

Cut down on omega-6 fats

Try to minimize your intake of vegetable oils that are rich in omega-6 essential fatty acids, such as sunflower and safflower oil, which promote inflammation in the body. Switch to olive oil for cooking, and macadamia nut oil or walnut oil for salad dressings (these are rich in healthy monounsaturated fats).

Drink plenty of fluid

Drink 2 to 3 quarts fluid a day to maintain good hydration and flow of nutrients to your joints. Choose from water, soups, tea, and juices, rather than sugary soft drinks.

Try elimination diets

If following the above guidelines for a healthy diet doesn't help relieve your arthritis symptoms, your joint pains may be associated with a food intolerance. If this is the case, an elimination diet might help you identify your trigger foods so you can avoid them in future. (See pages 50–51 for more details.)

Eat superfoods and take supplements

A number of superfoods are especially beneficial for your joint health and you should include them in your daily diet—I review them on pages 54–57. Nutritional supplements are also helpful (see pages 58–63). I also suggest specific supplement regimes for you to follow in each of the programs in Part Three.

eating more antioxidants

Antioxidants are beneficial substances found mainly in fruit, vegetables, tea, and wine. They include vitamins C and E, carotenoids, polyphenols, and the mineral selenium.

Why antioxidants are important

Arthritis is an inflammatory condition linked with the production of excess free radicals within the joints. Free radicals are unstable molecular fragments generated by normal metabolic reactions, exposure to environmental pollutants, doing exercise, smoking cigarettes, drinking alcohol, bathing in UVA sunlight, and taking certain drugs, especially antibiotics, and painkillers, such as aspirin. Free radicals are harmful because they carry a negative electrical charge in the form of a spare electron. They try to lose this negative charge by colliding with other molecules and cell structures in an attempt to neutralize it, either by passing on their spare electron, or by stealing a positive charge. This process is called oxidation. A good example of oxidation is the open-air interaction of iron with oxygen and water, to form rust.

Each cell in your body undergoes an estimated 10,000 free-radical oxidations a day, which trigger chain reactions in which spare electrical charges are shunted from one chemical to another, damaging proteins, fats, cartilage, cell membranes, and even genetic material.

Although you can't avoid generating a certain number of free radicals, you can help your joints by minimizing the amount of damage they do. Your main defense against free-radical attack is to consume as many antioxidants as possible. Antioxidants quickly mop up and neutralize the negative charges on free radicals before they can trigger a chain reaction.

Rating foods for antioxidant potential

To evaluate the antioxidant potential of different foods, scientists have developed a test called the Oxygen Radical Absorbance Capacity (ORAC; see box below). This shows how well the antioxidants present in fruits and vegetables can mop up the harmful free radicals that contribute to inflammatory processes in the body, such as arthritis (and that also contribute to premature aging).

Eating more antioxidants

The amount and types of fruit and vegetables you eat have a major impact on the level of inflammation in your joints. Different foods contain different types and amounts of antioxidants of varying potency.

What is the ORAC test?

The ORAC test measures how well the antioxidants in fruit and vegetables can block the breakdown of a chemical (fluorescein) after it's mixed with a strongly oxidant substance (peroxyl radical). Fluorescein is used because it's luminescent, and the intensity of light it emits decreases as it breaks down. This makes it easy to measure how much fluorescein remains intact at set intervals after being in contact with the oxidant and the fruit or vegetable extract. If the food has a low ORAC value, it provides little protection, fluorescein quickly breaks down and the mixture's luminosity decreases. If the food has a high ORAC value, it protects the fluorescein from degradation and the sample remains luminescent for much longer. After measuring the intensity of fluorescence in the mixture every 35 minutes after adding the oxidant, scientists compare the results with those obtained when using different concentrations of a standard antioxidant (trolox). Results are given in units known as "trolox equivalents," or TE.

The average person eating a typical Western diet eats just two-and-a-half portions of fruit and vegetables a day, which provides an estimated 5,700 ORAC units. Ideally, you need to obtain at least 7,000 ORAC units a day for good health. People who consume nine servings of fruit and vegetables a day can obtain as many as 20,000 ORAC units daily, which significantly reduce the amount of free-radical damage occurring within their joints.

As well as eating plenty of servings, you also need to make informed decisions about which fruit and vegetables you eat. For example, if you eat a kiwifruit, some watermelon, a mixed salad, and some cauliflower and carrots, you would obtain fewer than 2,000 ORAC units—even though you have achieved the recommended five servings a day. On the other hand, if you eat blueberries, plums, red kidney beans, spinach, and red bell peppers, you can rack up an astonishing 33,000 ORAC units in a single day. A number of herbs and spices have a surprisingly high ORAC score, too, even though you eat them only in small amounts. The higher your daily ORAC score, the higher your ability to neutralize free-radical damage to cells throughout your body, including your joints.

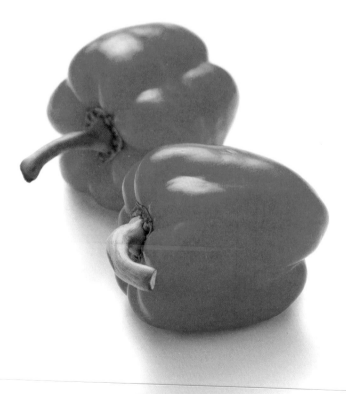

ORAC scores for herbs and spices

The following table provides you with the ORAC values for a range of herbs and spices (per gram). Adding just one gram of black pepper to a meal gives you an additional 301 ORAC units, while adding a gram of cinnamon supplies an amazing 2,675 ORAC units.

spice/herb	ORAC score* per gram
Cloves	3,144
Cinnamon	2,675
Oregano	2,001
Turmeric	1,592
Nutmeg	1,572
Cumin	768
Parsley	743
Basil leaf	676
Saffron	530
Curry powder	485
Sage leaf	320
Black peppercorns	301
Mustard seed	292
Ginger powder	288
Thyme	274
Cayenne pepper	236
Paprika	179
Mint	139
Garlic	54

*ORAC score = micromol of TE.

ORAC scores for a range of foods

This chart ranks a variety of foods (mostly fruit and vegetables) in terms of their ORAC score. The foods with the highest antioxidant potential per average serving are at the top.

food	ORAC score* per 3½ oz.	average serving size	ORAC score* per average serving	food	ORAC score* per 3½ oz.	average serving size	ORAC score* per average serving
Bittersweet chocolate	103,971	1½ oz.	41,588	Green peas (boiled)	4,039	⅓ cup	2,015
Lowbush blueberries	9,260	1 cup	13,427	Red grapes	1,260	32	2,016
Red kidney beans (raw)	14,413	½ cup	13,259	Red grapefruit	1,548	½ fruit	1,904
Pinto beans (raw)	12,359	½ cup	11,864	Beet (raw)	2,774	½ cup	1,886
Pomegranate	10,500	3½ oz.	10,500	Peaches (canned halves)	1,863	½ fruit	1,826
Cranberries	9,456	1 cup	8,983	Green grapes	1,118	32	1,789
Blackberries	5,348	1 cup	7,701	Mangoes (sliced)	1,002	1 cup	1,653
Red lentils (raw)	9,766	⅓ cup	7,325	Tangerines	1,620	1 med.	1,361
Prunes (dried)	8,578	½ cup	7,291	Pineapple (chopped)	793	1 cup	1,229
Globe artichoke	6,552	3½ oz.	6,552	Almonds (whole kernels)	4,454	22 nuts	1,265
Raspberries	4,925	1 cup	6,058	Onions (yellow, chopped)	1,220	⅔ cup	1,281
Strawberries (sliced)	3,577	1 cup	5,938	Red leaf lettuce	1,785	4 leaves	1,213
Red Delicious apple	4,275	1 small	5,900	Sweet potatoes (boiled)	766	1 med.	1,195
Pecan nuts (halves)	17,940	19 nuts	5,095	Radishes (sliced)	954	1 cup	1,107
Cherries (pitted)	3,361	1 cup	4,873	Red bell peppers (raw)	901	1 med.	1,072
Plums (black)	7,339	1 fruit	4,844	Spinach (raw)	2640	4 leaves	1,056
Russet potatoes (baked)	1,555	1 large	4,649	Eggplant (raw, cubed)	2,533	½ cup	1,039
Black beans (raw)	8,040	¼ cup	4,181	Bananas	879	1 med.	1,037
Plums (red)	6,239	1 fruit	4,118	Nectarines	749	1 med.	1,019
Gala apples	2,828	1 fruit	3,903	Broccoli (boiled, chopped)	1,259	½ cup	982
Walnuts (halves)	13,541	14 nuts	3,846	Peanuts	3,166	3 tbsp.	899
Golden Delicious apples	2,670	1 fruit	3,685	Carrots (raw)	1,215	1 med.	741
Dates	3,895	10 fruit	3,467	Kiwifruit (peeled)	918	1 fruit	698
Lemons/limes (sections)	2,412	⅔ cup	3,378	Green bell peppers (raw)	558	1 med.	664
Avocado (pitted, cubed)	1,933	1¼ cups	3,344	Corn (boiled)	728	1 ear	561
Pears (green, cubed)	1,911	1 cup	3,172	Pumpkin (raw, cubed)	483	1 cup	560
Chickpeas (raw)	4,030	¾ cup	3,022	Tomatoes (cooked)	460	½ cup	552
Pears (Red Anjou, cubed)	1,773	1 cup	2,943	Macadamia nuts	1,695	11 nuts	481
Hazelnuts	9,645	20 nuts	2,739	Green cabbage (boiled)	1,359	¼ cup	476
Navy beans (raw)	2,474	½ cup	2,573	Tomatoes (raw)	337	1 med.	415
Oranges (navel)	1,814	1 fruit	2,540	Lemon juice	1263	2 tbsp.	379
Figs	3,383	1½ med.	2,537	Cauliflower (raw)	647	½ cup	324
Raisins (packed cup)	3,037	½ cup	2,490	Watermelon (diced)	142	1 cup	216
Red cabbage (boiled)	3,146	½ cup	2,359	Lime juice	856	2 tbsp.	194
Red potatoes (baked)	1,326	1 med.	2,294	Carrots (cooked)	371	1 med.	171
Pistachios	7,983	49 nuts	2,267	Iceberg lettuce	451	2 leaves	144
Cowpeas (raw)	4,343	5 tbsp.	2,258	Cucumber (unpeeled)	115	½ cup	60

eliminating trigger foods

A number of foods have the potential to trigger joint pain in people with arthritis. Research shows that when avoiding foods that provoke symptoms, about 70 percent of people with all types of arthritis feel either better or much better, and report less pain, fewer painful joints, shorter duration of morning stiffness, and improved mobility and grip strength.

Identifying problem foods

How do you know which food or food groups—if any —you have a sensitivity to? The traditional way to find out is to follow an elimination-and-challenge diet (see below). This is time consuming, however, and people often find it difficult to comply with the strict dietary guidelines. A number of alternative tests can help identify problem foods; most are available only privately, such as via a naturopath.

The elimination-and-challenge diet This involves following a bland, hypoallergenic diet that includes only a few, limited foods considered least likely to result in joint inflammation, such as:

- Grains: white rice and tapioca.
- Fruit: pears and cranberries.
- Vegetables: squash, carrots, parsnips, lettuce, lentils, and split peas.
- Meat: wild game and turkey.

After 10 days of eating this bland diet, you then start to re-introduce eliminated foods, one by one, usually at three-day intervals. You keep a comprehensive food-and-symptom diary as you do this so you can see which foods cause your joint symptoms to flare up. If you notice a link between a specific food and a worsening in your symptoms, you should avoid that food and wait until your symptoms abate before testing another food. You can add any foods that don't trigger joint symptoms to the list of foods you can safely eat and enjoy in the future.

IgG blood tests A blood test that measures the levels of antibodies called IgG antibodies can identify the food/s to which you are intolerant. Your blood is subjected to sophisticated testing that identifies the presence of raised levels of IgG against more than 100 food antigens.

White blood cell analysis This test assesses how your white blood cells (leukocytes) react against specific food extracts. If your white blood cells don't respond to a specific food, it's unlikely to provoke your symptoms, and you can eat it freely. Foods that do activate your white blood cells, however, might

Your trigger foods

The foods most commonly found to worsen arthritis symptoms are: wheat, corn, rye, sugar, caffeine, yeast, malt, dairy products, oranges, grapefruit, lemons and tomatoes. The types of meats most likely to provoke symptoms are bacon, pork, beef and lamb. However, some of these foods are also arthritis superfoods and can actually help to improve joint health. Food intolerances are highly specific to the individual—culprit foods vary from one person to another. It's therefore important to keep a food-and-symptom diary to help pinpoint foods that provoke your symptoms. This is not always an easy task, as symptoms can sometimes worsen up to 36 hours after eating a trigger food.

provoke your arthritis, and you should avoid them initially—at least for five weeks—before re-introducing them, one by one, to see which, if any, are associated with joint flare-up. Research suggests this approach can improve arthritis symptoms in as many as 83 percent of cases.

Eliminating nightshade plants

Some people with arthritis are sensitive to foods from the nightshade (Solanaceae) family of plants. These plants produce varying amounts of chemicals known as steroidal glycoalkaloids as part of their natural defense against insects, fungi, and bacteria.

Some members of the nightshade family, such as the tobacco plant, Datura (Angel's Trumpets), mandrake, and Belladonna (deadly nightshade), produce toxic amounts of these alkaloids. Consuming these can trigger headache, dizziness, nausea, vomiting, diarrhea, abdominal pain, heart rhythm abnormalities, dilated pupils, muscle twitching, and weakness. Other members of the nightshade family produce very small amounts of glycoalkaloids and are familiar dietary staples. Commonly eaten nightshade foods include: potatoes, tamarillo, tomatoes, Cape gooseberries, eggplants, sweet bell peppers, chili peppers, paprika, cayenne and all other types of pepper, except black pepper, which belongs to a different family. Unlike many other plant toxins, glycoalkaloids are not broken down or detoxified by cooking, baking, or frying, which does, in fact, concentrate them.

Why some people experience a flare-up in joint symptoms as a result of eating nightshade plants is not fully understood, but it's possible the glycoalkaloids might trigger joint inflammation through an immune system mechanism or by altering calcium metabolism in bone. Another possibility is the recent finding that glycoalkaloids have an adverse effect on intestinal permeability to increase gut leakiness. This might increase the presence of other food allergens in the circulation to which the immune system can mount a response. This mechanism has also been suggested as a cause or aggravator of inflammatory bowel disease, such as Crohn's disease and ulcerative colitis, autoimmune conditions that are often accompanied by an inflammatory type of arthritis.

If you want to try eliminating nightshade foods from your diet, be prepared to wait for an improvement in your joint symptoms. It takes more than 24 hours for ingested glycoalkaloids to be cleared from your body, and if you eat foods containing them every day, they can accumulate in your body. You will usually notice the beneficial effects of eliminating nightshade foods within two to three weeks.

Research dating back to 1979 suggests eliminating nightshade foods from the diet improves arthritis symptoms in more than 70 percent of people with osteoarthritis, rheumatoid arthritis, and other joint problems. I explain how to eliminate nightshade foods in the moderate program (see pages 110–131).

Eliminating meat

Population studies have shown an association between the amount of meat fat, meat, and variety meat consumed in a country and the number of people with an inflammatory type of arthritis. Several studies have also suggested that eating a vegan or lactovegetarian diet can reduce the number of tender and swollen joints and shorten the duration of morning stiffness in people with rheumatoid arthritis.

Inflammatory arthritis is associated with intestinal inflammation, increased gut permeability, and raised levels of antibodies directed against gut bacteria and food antigens. Researchers have found similarities in the amino acid make-up of a cow protein (bovine albumin) and human collagen (present in joint cartilage).

It's possible that if the body mounts an immune response to eating beef, the antibodies intended to attack cow protein might attack human joints, too.

Switching to a lactovegetarian or vegan diet can also help joint symptoms by normalizing the pattern of bacteria present in the gut and improving the number of probiotic bacteria. The pattern of bacteria found in the bowel of people with early rheumatoid arthritis is significantly different from that in healthy people without rheumatoid arthritis. An abnormal pattern of bowel bacteria might result in the production of chemicals that increase joint inflammation.

Another advantage of eating a vegetarian diet is that you're likely to have an increased intake of anti-inflammatory antioxidants, including alphacarotene, betacarotene, lycopene, lutein, vitamin C, and vitamin E. This alone can improve joint health.

Eliminating "acid" foods

It's possible, for a reason that isn't yet understood, that foods classified as "acid" increase joint inflammation. In fact, the advice given by some naturopaths to people with arthritis is to eat a diet consisting of 60 to 80 percent alkaline foods and 20 to 40 percent acid foods.

There's a lot of confusion around the terms "acid" and "alkaline." They refer to the effects certain foods have on the pH of your urine—not whether the food itself is acidic or alkaline in quality, and not the effect it has on the acidity of your digestive system or even your blood. This is because your body works hard to keep the fluids bathing your cells within a very tight pH range of 7.35–7.45, which is slightly alkaline. If your blood pH falls even slightly outside of this range, you will become very ill. This is because your metabolism relies on a constant, low level of alkalinity to work properly.

When food is broken down, its various building blocks—proteins, carbohydrates, and fats—are metabolized to result in either the production or the consumption of varying amounts of protons. These are positively charged hydrogen ions (H+), the concentration of which determines the pH of a fluid. If the metabolism of a food results in the production of excess protons, it's classified as an acid food ("acid-forming" is a more accurate description). If the metabolism of a food uses up more protons than it produces, then it's classified as an alkaline (or alkaline-forming) food.

So, although some foods like oranges, lemons, limes, and tomatoes are acid to taste, the way their building blocks are metabolized in your body means they are classified as alkaline foods. Fruit is, in fact, your main dietary source of alkali. In contrast, protein-rich foods, such as meat and dairy products, are acid-forming. As amino acids, the building blocks of protein, are broken down, excess protons are produced. Your body gets rid of the acidity in the form of acidic carbon dioxide gas exhaled via your lungs, but some excess acid is also voided in your urine.

Not everyone is sensitive to acid-forming foods. If you can tolerate aspirin without experiencing a worsening in joint symptoms, then you're unlikely to have a problem with acid-forming foods. I don't recommend that you limit your intake of acid-forming

Vegan diets
As a vegan diet is associated with reduced intakes of vitamins B12 and D, people switching to a vegan diet should consider taking a vitamin-B12 supplement and, if sun exposure is limited, a vitamin-D supplement, too.

foods until you have tried other therapeutic dietary approaches (see Part Three) first. If you've done this and you still haven't got adequate symptom relief, try limiting acid-forming foods under the supervision of a qualified medical nutritionist. Many acid-forming foods are also important sources of protein, vitamins, minerals, and antioxidants. A medical nutritionist can tell you how to how best to replace these in your diet.

Eliminating purine-rich foods

Gout is a type of inflammatory arthritis that's caused by high levels of uric acid in joints and tissues. Uric acid comes from the breakdown of substances called purines in the body. Most of the uric acid we produce comes from the breakdown of purines that are released when the genetic material (DNA) of worn-out cells is recycled. However, some foods also contain purines, and changing your diet to eliminate purines can lower uric acid levels in your body by up to 20 percent. The following foods are rich in purines and you should avoid them if you have gout:

- Shellfish and oily fish
- Variety meat, meat, and game
- Yeast extract
- Asparagus
- Spinach

I also suggest that you avoid alcohol. It both increases uric-acid production and reduces its excretion. Cut out beer, especially, which is very rich in purines.

Acid- and alkaline-forming foods

Acid-forming foods

Vegetables with a high protein or sulfur content: grains (barley, oats, quinoa, rice, wheat); legumes (for example, black beans, chickpeas, kidney beans, lentils, and soybeans), most nuts (pecans, cashews, peanuts, pistachios, and walnuts)

Some fruits: blueberries, cranberries, plums, prunes

Dairy products: cheese, milk, ice cream, yogurt

Animal proteins: eggs, poultry, meat, seafood

Alcohol: beer, wine

Alkaline-forming foods

Mildly alkaline: low-sugar fruit, such as sour cherries; berries; grapefruit; lemons; limes; bell peppers

Strongly alkaline: green leafy vegetables, such as kale, broccoli, and spinach; avocado; tomato

superfoods for arthritis

The food and drinks in this chart have a natural anti-inflammatory action that's particularly beneficial for people with arthritis. Try to incorporate at least five of these superfoods into your diet every day. However, avoid foods that trigger an idiosyncratic reaction and worsen your arthritis.

superfood	benefits	how to use it
Apples Contain anti-inflammatory antioxidants and bone-friendly boron and magnesium. Red Delicious apples contain the most antioxidants in their skin and flesh.	Eating even an extra-small apple provides the same antioxidant benefits for inflamed joints as 1,500 mg vitamin C. Wash, but don't peel your apples—the antioxidants are five times more concentrated in the skin than the flesh.	Eat as a daily snack. Grate (mix with lemon juice to prevent browning) and add to salads and coleslaw. Eat dried apple rings and apple chips. Cloudy apple juice has more antioxidants than clear.
Avocado Contains antioxidant monounsaturated oils, essential fatty acids, beta-sitosterol, and vitamin E.	Avocado can suppress joint inflammation by reducing production of inflammatory substances. It promotes cartilage repair in osteoarthritis by stimulating the activity of bone-building cells and cartilage cells.	Eat as an appetizer and add to salads. Mash to make dips, such as guacamole, or simply spread onto oat crackers.
Brazil nuts The richest dietary source of selenium—a single Brazil nut contains about 50 mcg. Selenium improves the quality of cartilage proteins. Also a good source of magnesium and sulfur.	People with the highest dietary intake of selenium are least likely to develop osteoarthritis. Each increase of 0.1 parts per million of selenium in your toenail clippings (a good indicator of selenium status) lowers your risk of knee osteoarthritis by 20 percent.	Eat as a snack. Scatter cereal over, yogurts, and salads. Brazil nut butter is a delicious spread. Buy little and often for maximum freshness.
Chili peppers Contain substances called capsaicin and dihydrocapsaicin.	Capsaicin and dihydrocapsaicin block transmission of pain messages. They also trigger the release of endorphins—the brain's own morphinelike painkillers. Capsaicin is used in clinical trials as a long-acting analgesic to treat post-surgical and osteoarthritis pain. A single injection at the site of pain acts for several months.	Add chili peppers to curries, soups, and stews. Use sweet chili jelly as a conserve with meats and cheeses.

superfood	benefits	how to use it
Curry powder spices For example, anise, chili, cloves, cumin, fennel, ginger, mustard, and turmeric.	Curry spices have a painkilling, anti-inflammatory action that helps to alleviate joint symptoms. Mustard isothiocyanates reduce inflammation in a similar way to aspirin. Turmeric and ginger contain curcumin, which can reduce cartilage destruction in osteoarthritis, and prevent the onset of rheumatoid arthritis.	Increase your consumption of spiced Indian and Middle Eastern foods.
Dark green leafy vegetables For example, broccoli, spinach, spring greens, dark green cabbage, and parsley. These vegetables supply antioxidant carotenoids, vitamin C, calcium, and magnesium.	A high antioxidant diet is good for arthritis (see pages 47–49). Sixty-one percent of the bone-friendly calcium found in broccoli is absorbed from the gut, compared with only 32 percent of calcium in milk. (The reason for this remains unknown.)	Steam greens lightly to accompany meals. Use raw baby spinach leaves in salads. Add leaves to the mixture when juicing fruit and vegetables.
Dark blue-red pigmented fruits For example, cherries, grapes, blueberries, bilberries, dark raspberries, and elderberries. These contain antioxidant anthocyanins.	Anthocyanins lower levels of inflammatory chemicals in the body. Eating just 9 ounces dark red cherries daily can lower uric acid levels enough to prevent gout. Drinking a glass of red grape juice has an antioxidant action that lasts for two hours after ingestion.	Eat fresh or frozen. Add to yogurt, muesli, fromage blanc, fruit salads, or any other dessert. Puree to make a coulis. Juice berries and dilute with apple juice for a refreshing, antioxidant-rich drink.
Garlic Contains beneficial substances, such as allicin.	A Russian study has shown that people with rheumatoid arthritis can benefit from increasing the amount of garlic they eat.	Add to all savory dishes just before the end of cooking.
Grapefruit Contains vitamin C and antioxidant bioflavonoids. Red grapefruit has a higher antioxidant content than yellow grapefruit.	Grapefruit helps to reduce inflammation, strengthen cartilage, and block prostaglandins (substances involved in pain). It increases the anti-inflammatory effect of some painkillers. Eating grapefruit regularly improves symptoms in some people with rheumatoid and other forms of inflammatory arthritis.	Eat as an appetizer; add to fruit salads; drink the freshly squeezed juice. Check for drug interactions with the pharmacist who dispenses your usual prescriptions.
Macadamias The richest food source of monounsaturated fatty acids and an excellent source of vitamin E and selenium.	The antioxidant action reduces inflammation in arthritis. The nuts are being used in a trial to reduce the risk of rheumatoid arthritis.	Eat a handful as a snack; scatter over cereal, yogurts, and salads. Macadamia nut butter is a delicious spread.

superfood	benefits	how to use it
Milk A good source of calcium and B-vitamins.	People who drink milk daily are significantly less likely to have clinical or x-ray evidence of knee osteoarthritis than those with a lower consumption (after taking other dietary factors into account).	Pour over cereals for breakfast; add to drinks such as tea; and use to make smoothies, shakes, and milk puddings.
Mushrooms Medicinal mushrooms such as *Tricholoma giganteum*, reishi (*Ganoderma lucidum*), maitake (*Grifola frondosa*), and *Phellinus linteus* contain immune-modulating substances.	Medicinal mushrooms can inhibit production of inflammatory substances in experimental models of arthritis.	Slice into salads; make into soup; sauté in olive oil with garlic; bake stuffed with mashed butternut squash and parsley. Take reishi or maitake supplements.
Oily fish A rich source of anti-inflammatory omega-3 fatty acids (EPA and DHA).	A large analysis of 17 studies assessing the pain-relieving effects of omega-3 fatty acids in rheumatoid and other autoimmune forms of arthritis showed they significantly reduce joint pain and intensity, the duration of morning stiffness, the number of painful joints, and the need to take NSAID painkillers—all within three to four months.	Eat fish that's as fresh as possible, and preferably raw, such as sushi and sashimi, or steamed, broiled, or baked until just set. Eat two to four portions of oily fish a week—girls and women who might get pregnant in the future should limit their intake to two portions a week to reduce their exposure to mercury.
Olive oil A rich source of monounsaturated fats, and antioxidant, anti-inflammatory substances.	Increased olive oil consumption is associated with a reduced risk of rheumatoid arthritis and cardiovascular disease. Olive oil might protect against the development of osteoarthritis.	Use plain olive oil for cooking. Use extra virgin olive oil (made from the first pressing of the olives) in salad dressings and for drizzling on food. (It has the highest antioxidant content, but smokes at high heat.)
Onions A rich source of quercetin, an antioxidant bioflavonoid that suppresses the production of inflammatory substances. Red onions are particularly high in antioxidants.	Quercetin binds to cartilage and strengthens its structure. As an antioxidant it mops up free radicals within joints and reduces the release of protein-degrading enzymes.	Make French onion soup. Serve onion sauces and onion marmalade with meat dishes. Slice raw red onions into salads.
Pomegranate A rich source of antioxidant polyphenols, anthocyanins, vitamins C and E, and carotenoids. Its antioxidant potential is two or three times higher than that of red wine and green tea.	Ellagic acid in pomegranate juice reduces inflammation by blocking activation of inflammatory substances that play a key role in cartilage degradation in osteoarthritis.	Buy fresh pomegranate juice drinks or make your own. Add pomegranate seeds to salads and desserts.

superfood	benefits	how to use it
Red wine A rich source of antioxidant polyphenols, such as resveratrol.	Resveratrol blocks the release of inflammatory substances, which helps to reduce joint inflammation.	Drink one or two glasses, once or twice a week (as long as wine doesn't worsen your arthritis symptoms).
Soybeans These contain antioxidant isoflavones that have a beneficial estrogenlike action to strengthen bones.	Soy suppresses joint inflammation and pain. It blocks production of inflammatory substances in joints and promotes the repair of cartilage in osteoarthritis by stimulating the activity of osteoblasts (bone-building cells) and chondrocytes (cartilage cells).	Use soybeans in soups, stews, and stir-fries. Use tofu and soy sauce in cooking. Add soybean protein powder to shakes.
Teas White, green, oolong, and black teas contain high levels of antioxidant catechins, such as epigallocatechin-3-gallate (EGCG).	EGCG inhibits the expression of inflammatory mediators in arthritic joints and helps to protect cartilage degradation in osteoarthritis.	Drink green, black, or white tea regularly, three to five times a day. Use leftover cold tea to soak dried fruit. Use green or white tea as a basis for sauces, soups, or stews or to make ice cream.
Walnuts A rich source of omega-3 fatty acids.	Omega-3 fatty acids have an anti-inflammatory action. Some research shows that eating walnuts daily can help alleviate the symptoms of rheumatoid arthritis.	Add chopped walnuts to cereals, salads, vegetarian dishes, and desserts. Use walnut butter as a spread.
Yellow or orange fruit and vegetables For example, carrots, sweet potatoes, guava, mango, and pumpkin—these are all rich sources of vitamin C and antioxidant carotenoids.	Fruit and vegetables with a high antioxidant content can reduce pain and inflammation in all types of arthritis.	Eat fresh in fruit salads or on its own for dessert. Puree to make fruit coulis, shakes, and smoothies. Dried mango makes a deliciously healthy sweet snack (avoid those preserved with sulftes).
Yogurt with live cultures Contains probiotic bacteria.	Probiotic bacteria help to reduce the severity of joint inflammation. They also reduce abnormal intestinal bacterial balance (dysbiosis) associated with "leakiness" of the gut wall and food intolerance.	Eat lowfat yogurt with live cultures with breakfast cereals, and with chopped fruit in desserts. Drink probiotic yogurt drinks.

supplements for arthritis

These are the supplements that I believe are of most benefit to your joint health. They also help to alleviate the symptoms of both osteoarthritis and autoimmune arthritis. Whereas prescribed drugs such as NSAIDs (see pages 19–20) can only damp down inflammation and pain, some supplements, such as glucosamine and chondroitin, have the potential to halt the degenerative changes of osteoarthritis.

Each supplement tends to be effective for two out of three people with joint pain, so choose a supplement and try it for a couple of months until you find one that works for you. Most joint health supplements can be taken together for additional, synergistic benefits. As well as being as effective as some prescribed analgesics, supplements are less likely to cause adverse side effects.

supplement	research findings	dose and comments
Vitamin B5 (pantothenic acid) This is vital for many energy-producing reactions in the body. It also stimulates cell growth in healing tissues. Vitamin B5 is rapidly depleted during times of stress.	Lack of B5 causes defects in cartilage formation. Blood levels of B5 are lower than normal in people with rheumatoid arthritis. When people with rheumatoid arthritis were given B5 injections, symptoms improved in most cases, but recurred when supplementation was discontinued. Oral supplements of calcium pantothenate can reduce the duration of morning stiffness, degree of disability, and severity of pain in rheumatoid arthritis.	An intake of 4–7 mg is believed to be adequate. Nutritional therapists might prescribe higher doses of 50–200 mg daily.
Vitamin B6 Needed to lower levels of homocysteine—a harmful, inflammatory amino acid that can cause hardening and furring up of the arteries (atherosclerosis).	People with rheumatoid arthritis have low B6-levels, raised homocysteine levels, and an increased risk of heart disease. Vitamin B6 can help alleviate carpal tunnel syndrome (CTS), which can affect people with osteoarthritis of the wrist. It can also reduce hand pain in osteoarthritis.	An intake of 2 mg daily is believed to be adequate. Nutritional therapists might prescribe higher doses of 10–200 mg daily.

supplement	research findings	dose and comments
Folate (Vitamin B9) Needed to lower homocysteine levels.	Can reduce hand pain in osteoarthritis by reducing systemic inflammation.	The normal optimum intake is 400 mcg daily. Nutritional therapists recommend 400–1,000 mcg daily. Folic acid—the synthetic form of folate—is more easily absorbed and used in the body than the naturally occurring folate. Folic acid should usually be taken together with vitamin B12 to avoid masking B12 deficiency.
Vitamin B12 Needed to lower homocysteine levels.	Levels of vitamin B12 tend to be low in people with rheumatoid arthritis, psoriatic arthropathy, and lupus, and this contributes to a high incidence of anemia (35–49 percent in these groups).	The usual recommended intake is 1 mcg daily. Nutritional therapists recommend up to 1,000 mcg daily.
Vitamin C (ascorbic acid) This is a powerful antioxidant. It's needed for the production of collagen in ligaments and cartilage.	Lack of vitamin C can contribute to cartilage aging. Vitamin C-supplements can reduce hip and knee pain as a result of osteoarthritis. In a study of 640 men and women, those with moderate to high intakes of vitamin C (two or more times the recommended dietary allowance) were three times less likely to develop knee pain or see their knee osteoarthritis progress than those with a lower intake of vitamin C (up to about twice the recommended daily amount).	The usual recommended intake is 60–120 mg daily. Nutritional therapists recommend up to 1–3 g daily. Vitamin C supplements can cause indigestion—to overcome this, use ester-C, a nonacidic form that is more readily absorbed and used in the body.
Vitamin D This is essential for the absorption of dietary calcium and phosphate in the small intestine, and for the deposition of calcium and phosphate in bone, and for bone modeling. It can be synthesized in the body by the action of sunlight (UVB rays) on the skin.	Cartilage and bone is sensitive to lack of vitamin D. In people with low vitamin-D levels, osteoarthritis of the hip is more likely. Osteoarthritis can progress three to four times more rapidly in some people with vitamin D deficiency. Vitamin D supplements can relieve joint pain in some people with osteoarthritis. People with low vitamin-D levels are also 33 percent more likely to develop rheumatoid arthritis.	The usual recommended intake is 5–10 mcg. Up to 25 mcg daily isn't thought to be harmful.

supplement	research findings	dose and comments
Vitamin E This is a powerful antioxidant.	Vitamin E blocks the action of inflammatory prostaglandins to relieve pain. It also helps to stabilize joint cartilage. People with the highest intake of vitamin E are half as likely to develop osteoarthritis of the knee as those with the lowest intakes. Research shows that vitamin E can be twice as effective as a placebo or simple analgesics in reducing pain levels in some people with osteoarthritis. Low vitamin-E levels appear to increase the risk of developing rheumatoid arthritis.	The usual recommeneded intake is 10 mg daily. Nutritional therapists might prescribe higher doses of up to 727 mg (800 IU) daily. Take together with vitamin C, which is needed to regnerae vitamin E.
Boron A trace mineral that plays a role in bone calcium metabolism by boosting production of the active form of vitamin D.	Bone boron levels are lower than normal in people with arthritis. In areas where boron intakes are low (less than or equal to 1 mg daily), the incidence of arthritis ranges from 20–70 percent, but where boron intakes are good (3–10 mg daily), the incidence of arthritis is 10 percent or less. Boron appears to protect against both osteoarthritis and rheumatoid arthritis, but the mechanism remains unknown.	A daily intake of 3 mg is suggested as optimum for bone health. Nutritional therapists might prescribe higher doses of 3–9 mg per day as part of a multivitamin and mineral supplement.
Calcium A mineral that is vital for the maintenance of strong, healthy bones.	People with arthritis have reduced mobility and are at risk of future osteoporosis, especially if their intake of calcium is low and/or they take corticosteroids. Calcium supplements can improve bone strength in people with all types of arthritis.	Intakes of 800–1,000 mg are needed for optimal bone health. Nutritional therapists might prescribe doses of 300–1,500 mg. High doses should usually be taken together with other minerals, such as zinc, iron, and magnesium. Calcium tablets are best taken with meals. People who tend to suffer from kidney stones should take calcium supplements together with essential fatty acids (ask your doctor about this).
Magnesium A mineral that is important for the action of virtually all body enzymes, and for maintaining the integrity of cells.	People with rheumatoid arthritis tend to have low magnesium levels and reduced activity of this enzyme. Low levels of magnesium contribute to fatigue.	300mg daily. Make sure you maintain a good calcium intake when you take magnesium supplements.

supplement	research findings	dose and comments
Selenium A trace element needed to make powerful antioxidant enzymes (glutathione peroxidases) that reduce inflammation in the body. Selenium also increases the effectiveness of vitamin E.	Lack of selenium is associated with greater severity of osteoarthritis and rheumatoid arthritis.	Intakes of about 75 mcg are believed to be adequate. Nutritional therapists might recommend doses of 50–200 mcg. Selenium that's organically bound to yeast is more readily absorbed and usable than selenium salts.
Zinc An essential trace element needed for the action of over a hundred different enzymes. It helps to regulate gene activation and the synthesis of specific proteins.	People with rheumatoid arthritis tend to have a reduced ability to absorb zinc, and a lower than normal zinc level. Supplements supplying zinc sulfate appear to have a beneficial disease-modifying action in psoriatic arthropathy, and to reduce the need for painkillers.	15mg daily.
Evening primrose oil A source of an anti-inflammatory omega-6 essential fatty acid called gammalinolenic acid (GLA).	Research shows that taking evening primrose oil for three months might enable people with rheumatoid arthritis to reduce their dose of NSAID painkillers. Evening primrose oil can also reduce fatigue in people with autoimmune conditions, such as rheumatoid arthritis.	Take 500 mg to 3 g daily. This is equivalent to 40 mg and 240 mg GLA. Do not take evening primrose oil if you have a rare disorder known as temporal lobe epilepsy.
Omega-3 fish oils A rich source of omega-3 fatty acids, EPA, and DHA (eicosapentaenoic acid and docosahexaenoic acid).	EPA and DHA damp down inflammation and can reduce the long-term need for painkillers in people with joint pain. They might also reduce the risk of coronary heart disease in people with rheumatoid arthritis.	Take 500 mg to 4 g daily. For severe inflammatory disease, nutritional therapists might recommend up to 6 g daily. Fish oils can cause belching and mild nausea. Seek medical advice before taking fish-oil supplements if you have a blood-clotting disorder or are taking a blood-thinning drug, such as aspirin or warfarin. (Fish oils can increase the tendency to bleed.) If you have diabetes, monitor your glucose levels carefully when taking fish-oil supplements.
Cod liver oil (CLO) Contains omega-3 essential fatty acids and vitamins A and D.	Cod liver oil can reduce the intensity of musculoskeletal pain. It can also reduce the incidence of gastrointestinal side effects produced by NSAID therapy.	Take a supplement described as "extra high strength" or "concentrated." Do not take cod liver oil supplements during pregnancy.

nutritional approaches to treatment

supplement	research findings	dose and comments
Green-lipped mussel extracts Contain an omega-3 fatty acid (eicosatetraenoic acid) that inhibits the production of a group of inflammatory substances in the body.	Green-lipped mussel extracts reduce arthritis symptoms more than NSAIDs, such as ibuprofen or indomethacin. A study published in 2003 found these extracts significantly improved the signs and symptoms of osteoarthritis by 53 percent within one month, and 80 percent within two months. A clinical trial involving 30 people with rheumatoid arthritis and 30 with osteoarthritis found significant benefit for 23 with the rheumatoid condition and 21 with osteoarthritis.	Take 200–1,200 mg daily. Supplements are available in powdered or oil form.
Glucosamine A natural substance needed for the repair of cartilage, but one that's often in short supply. It's used to both treat and prevent osteoarthritis.	Glucosamine sulfate supplements can improve osteoarthritis symptoms by as much as 73 percent and are at least as effective as paracetamol in reducing pain. A trial published in *The Lancet* (2001) concluded taking 1,500 mg glucosamine daily produced significant improvements in pain and disability in people with osteoarthritis of the knee, with no significant loss of joint space over the three-year trial period. And a systematic review of 20 trials found, in people with osteoarthritis, glucosamine was more effective at relieving pain than a placebo, with a 28 percent improvement in pain and a 21 percent improvement in joint function.	Take 1,000–2,000 mg daily. Glucosamine is often combined with other ingredients, such as chondroitin, selenium, or MSM to increase its effectiveness.
Chondroitin sulfate This attracts water into joints, which acts a shock absorber, as well as a nutrient transport system. It inhibits enzymes that break down cartilage, while stimulating those involved in the production of structural substances. It is used to treat osteoarthritis.	Research shows that taking chondroitin significantly improves pain and joint function in people with osteoarthritis of the knee within three months. In people taking a placebo, joint space width decreased, while in those taking chondroitin, there was no deterioration in joint space.	Take 800–1,600 mg daily. Chondroitin is often combined with glucosamine—the two supplements have a naturally synergistic action.

the natural health approach

supplement	research findings	dose and comments
MSM (methyl-sulphonyl-methane) A sulfur compound that has an anti-inflammatory action. It reduces the formation of free radicals by white blood cells.	MSM can reduce joint pain in people with osteoarthritis by 82 percent within six weeks, compared with an average improvement of 18 percent in those taking a placebo. The combination of 500 mg glucosamine plus 500 mg MSM three times a day can significantly improve joint function and reduce pain and swelling more than either supplement on its own. The combination also produces a more rapid improvement in symptoms.	Take 1–2 g daily, in divided doses. MSM is often taken together with glucosamine.
Garlic Provides allicin (diallyl thiosulfinate), which is a powerful antioxidant and a source of sulfur. It has an anti-inflammatory action related to that of MSM.	A Russian study has shown that 86 percent of people with rheumatoid arthritis who took a garlic supplement experienced a reduction in arthritis symptoms within four to six weeks, with no side effects.	Take 600–900 mg daily. Select tablets standardized to provide 1,000–1,500 mcg allicin. Choose products with an enteric coating, which reduces odor and protects active ingredients from degradation in the stomach.
Collagen hydrolysates These are essentially gelatin obtained from the carcasses of chickens, pigs, sheep, or cows. They provide building blocks, such as chondroitin sulfate for joint repair, and can reduce pain in those with severe symptoms of arthritis.	Collagen hydrolysates can help promote joint cartilage renewal. In a six-month study of 100 older people, those taking collagen hydrolysates showed significant improvement in joint mobility compared with those taking placebo.	Take 300 mg to 1 g daily.
CMO (cis-9-cetyl myristoleate) This is a waxy oil containing cetylated fatty acids. It acts as a joint lubricant and has an anti-inflammatory action. It's used to treat all types of arthritis.	CMO helps to lubricate joints and can reduce pain either when taken in oral form, or when rubbed onto a joint as a cream. Research has shown that 68 days of taking oral CMO can bring about a significant increase in the range of knee movement in people with osteoarthritis, improving flexion by 10 degrees.	Take 300–600 mg daily. You can take CMO with an enzyme (lipase), to aid its digestion. Tobacco, alcohol, and caffeine use are reported to reduce the effectiveness of CMO.

lifestyle approaches to treatment

Changing aspects of your lifestyle can bring about dramatic improvements in the way you feel. Something as basic as losing weight, for example, can relieve pressure on your joints and go a long way to easing pain and stiffness. It can also improve your mobility and boost your self-esteem. On the next few pages, I explain the most important adjustments you can make to your lifestyle in terms of relieving joint symptoms and maximizing joint health.

Quit smoking

Smoking is a risk factor for developing rheumatoid arthritis, and it increases disease activity and severity once you have rheumatoid arthritis. It also hastens the hardening and furring up of your arteries and has a more dangerous effect on artery walls in people with rheumatoid arthritis than in the general population. For people with osteoarthritis of the knee, smoking increases cartilage loss and is associated with more severe knee pain than in those who don't smoke. Some studies also suggest that smoking is associated with low-back pain. These effects might be related to blood-vessel constriction and a reduced supply of oxygen and nutrients to joints and intervertebral disks.

Drink in moderation

If you drink an excessive amount of alcohol, you're at an increased risk of developing rheumatoid arthritis. Alcohol is toxic to muscle cells and can also increase the risk of tendon rupture in people with inflammatory disease. If you're trying to lose weight, limiting your alcohol intake is an easy way to cut back on calories. Aim to drink no more than two or three units of alcohol a day.

Find ways to deal with stress

Prolonged stress lowers your pain threshold and increases your perception of joint pain. Stress can also increase disease activity in rheumatoid arthritis. Try to avoid stressful situations through forward planning and learn to say "no" when unreasonable demands are made on you. If you start to feel stressed, stop what you are doing, take a deep breath, and inwardly say "calm" to yourself. Try listening to calming music to help you unwind; and place a few drops of a flower essence, such as Rescue Remedy, under your tongue. Many of the complementary therapies in Part Two can reduce the effects of stress—try aromatherapy, yoga, qigong, massage, reflexology, acupressure, and meditation.

Choose a good mattress

Many people with arthritis sleep on a mattress that is too hard or too soft, and this can make joint pain worse. Scientists have now developed the perfect sleeping surface, a visco-elastic polymer that is heat and pressure sensitive and naturally molds to your body. This "memory foam" gives firm support as your body sinks comfortably into the material, supporting the natural curves of your back, reducing the load on pressure points, and helping muscles and ligaments recover during sleep. Reduction of strain on your pressure points also reduces the number of times you turn during sleep from 50 to 80 times a night to about 20 times. This lessens restlessness and pain, which, in turn, reduces the need for sleeping tablets and painkillers. See your local mattress supplier for details of brands such as Integra and Tempur.

Choose shoes that reduce joint stress

Exercise and weight loss can improve pain from knee arthritis, but until recently little attention was paid to the design of shoes. Masai Barefoot Technology (MBT) make shoes with a reverse heel that mimics walking on unstable ground. This forces you to walk more naturally, in an upright manner. MBT shoes dynamically alter weight loading so pressure is distributed evenly through your foot from the moment your heel strikes the ground to the moment your toes lift off. Research shows that wearing MBT shoes can reduce stress on knee and hip joints by about 20 percent, and increase muscle activity in your lower limbs and thigh muscles by a similar amount. Many osteopaths, chiropractors, physiotherapists, and orthopedic surgeons recommend MBT shoes to treat lower back pain and arthritis. The shoes are available in more than 20 countries and are classed as medical devices in the European Union. Trials show they can improve pain, stiffness, and physical functioning by at least 10 percent, with benefits occurring within the first three to six weeks.

Use a walking aid

Using a walking stick improves balance and more than halves the load on a damaged leg joint. If you have pain or weakness on one side, hold the stick in the opposite hand. So, for example, if your right leg is painful, use the stick in your left hand. When walking, start by putting all your weight on your stronger leg. Now step forward with your affected leg and the walking stick at the same time. This allows you to support your weight

Tips to help you quit smoking
- Find support—stopping smoking is much easier when you do it with a friend.
- Suck on artificial cigarettes or chew carrot sticks to help overcome cravings.
- Consider using nicotine replacement products or nicotine-trapping drops (available from drug stores) that you add to cigarette filters.
- Keep your hands busy—draw, knit, paint, or play with worry beads.

on a combination of your affected leg and the stick, so you can now step forward using your stronger leg. To walk upstairs, put your stronger leg on the first step, then bring your affected leg and the walking stick onto the same step. Repeat these actions, so you go up the steps one by one. To walk downstairs, start by lowering your bad leg and the walking stick onto the top step. Next, bring your better leg down onto that same step and continue going down one step at a time. Always keep your free hand on the railing.

If you're using a walking stick to help you balance, then use whichever hand makes you feel most comfortable and stable. Place the stick firmly on the ground and step forward only once you feel secure.

Use other lifestyle aids

A variety of assistive devices can make life more comfortable. For example, wedge a lumbar support between your seat and your lower back to make sitting easier. And wear a joint support around affected joints to keep them warm and stable. When traveling, support your head on a U-shaped travel pillow to mimimize jolts and to relieve neck pain; and use soft pillows on armrests.

doing regular exercise

Whatever form of arthritis you have, gentle exercise helps to maintain your joint mobility and function and provides reductions in pain and disability. Yet, many people with arthritis don't exercise because they fear it will make their joints worse.

The benefits of exercise

Researchers have found particular forms of exercise may have a positive effect on joint health in people with osteoarthritis and rheumatoid arthritis.

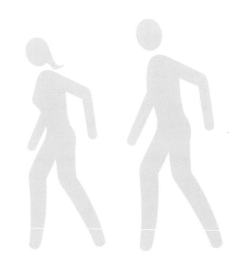

Osteoarthritis Exercise can postpone the onset of osteoarthritis or slow its progress if you already have it. When researchers from Stanford University, in California, compared 538 members of a running club with 423 people who never exercised, they found running offers up to 12 years protection against the onset of osteoarthritis. Those who ran between six and 20 miles a week gained the most benefit. All participants were aged around 58 and were assessed regularly for pain and disability, as well as having the progression of osteoarthritis checked using x-rays. Twenty percent of those who did do any exercise had pain and disability compared with only five percent of the runners, with women being at greatest risk of disability. Other studies suggest strength training might slow knee arthritis, and lower body exercises can reduce the rate of space narrowing in the knee joint.

Some researchers believe weight-bearing exercise, such as running, is helpful because it encourages the production of synovial fluid that helps lubricate the joints. Excessive running, however, can put joints under strain. Also, any sport that twists the joints, such as football or rugby, can cause tearing and injury, which

are risk factors for developing osteoarthritis, especially in the knee.

A study called the Fitness, Arthritis, and Seniors Trial (FAST) involved 435 people with knee osteoarthritis, aged 60 or over, and they were randomly assigned to an 18-month health-education program, a weight-training program, or an aerobic-exercise program. The participants who did aerobic exercise showed the biggest improvements in walking speed and the biggest reductions in pain and disability. Another study involving 100 people over the age of 60 who had knee arthritis showed that exercise—whether walking or weight training—improved stability and reduced the tendency to sway while standing. And for people with osteoarthritis of the hands, home exercises can help to protect the joints and can increase grip strength by 25 percent.

Rheumatoid arthritis If you're struggling to cope with both the pain and fatigue of rheumatoid arthritis, aerobic exercise might seem impossible. In the past people with rheumatoid arthritis were advised to do only nonweight-bearing, isometric exercises because of concerns that more intensive exercise might worsen pain and damage joints. We now know, however, aerobic exercise is the most helpful form of exercise. It not only improves your muscle strength and joint mobility, it also increases your cardiorespiratory fitness.

People with rheumatoid arthritis who exercise more than three times a week for at least 20 minutes have significantly less fatigue and disability after six months when compared with nonexercisers. And these benefits occur without any increase in pain and without any apparent worsening of disease activity or arthritis progression. Long-term, high-intensity, weight-bearing exercises might even have a protective effect on certain joints, such as those in the feet, and can slow down the loss of bone-mineral density at the hip.

However, this advice doesn't include all people with rheumatoid arthritis. If you have extensive damage to your large joints, high-intensity, weight-bearing exercises might accelerate the progression of joint damage. Instead, try a nonweight-bearing form of exercise, such as swimming. Research shows moderately intense swimming twice a week in a temperate hydrotherapy pool can significantly improve muscle function in both upper and lower extremities.

How much exercise?

People with all forms of arthritis should aim to exercise on at least five days a week, and preferably every day if possible. Your aim should be to start slowly, and gradually work up to 40 minutes exercise a day. You can then start increasing the intensity and/or duration of your exercise program.

You don't have to complete your daily exercise in a single session. If it makes it easier, do two or three shorter daily sessions of 10 to 15 minutes each.

Try to base your exercise schedule on the following:

- Do range-of-movement exercises every day to maintain and increase flexibility. This involves putting each joint through its full range of movement by bending, stretching, and extending it. I include suitable a stretch routine in the gentle program.
- Do muscle-strengthening exercises, using small weights, every other day.
- Do aerobic exercise at least three times a week—and every day if you can.

Types of exercise

Physical activity doesn't need to be vigorous, and it's important to find a type of exercise that you enjoy so you are motivated to keep it up long term. Even fun activities, such as doing home-handyman

Coping with discomfort

Pace yourself and respect your limitations when you exercise. Adjust your level of activity to your level of discomfort—if a joint becomes red, swollen or painful, ease off. Learn to listen to your body. If you feel worse the day after exercise, for example, you might have done too much or the activity you chose might not have been suitable for you. Find ways to minimize pain. Research suggests some people with arthritis suffer less pain for up to six hours after sexual intercourse. This might result from increased production of analgesic endorphins in the brain, or from increased secretion of hormones, such as testosterone, which have an anti-inflammatory effect. You can also try taking a painkiller before exercise to help relax your muscles and decrease the likelihood of spasm. In addition, you can apply a hot pack to sore joints before exercise. It will relieve pain, increases circulation, and relax muscles. If your joints are painful after exercise, apply an ice pack to them to reduce or prevent swelling and relieve pain.

projects, gardening, dancing, and sex, count as exercise.

Many people with arthritis are able to enjoy activities that involve weight-bearing, such as walking, golf, and bowling. You might even be able to do more intensive forms of exercise, such as gardening, dancing, or jogging. If walking is painful, however, try a less weight-bearing form of exercise, such as swimming or cycling (on a recumbent or stationary bike, if you prefer). If your arthritis is very advanced, then non-weight-bearing exercise, such as cycling or swimming, especially in a hydrotherapy pool (see page 30), is most appropriate.

Walking This is an excellent form of exercise. Invest in a good pair of walking shoes with cushioned soles and some ankle support to protect your feet and lower joints, and consider using a stick (see page 65). When walking, your feet should ideally turn out slightly (15 to 20 degrees) to provide optimum support, and be planted eight to 10 inches apart. Keep your knees slightly flexed, and avoid walking on the inner edges of your soles, because this makes your ankles rock inward and throws your body out of alignment. Try to keep your head up and keep your tummy and pelvis tucked in and your body tilted slightly forward so your weight is on the balls of your feet.

Cycling This is a low-impact, nonweight-bearing aerobic activity that, like swimming, doesn't put your muscles, ligaments or joints under excessive strain. You can cycle at home or in the gym on a stationary bike, or outdoors. Studies have shown that people who exercise in the fresh air derive greater benefits and get fitter more quickly than those who exercise indoors. Start cycling with a low-gear ratio to keep resistance low. As your stamina increases, introduce more intense bursts of exercise to increase your fitness,

if your joints allow. Maintain and oil your bike regularly, and wear a safety helmet made to a recognized standard. Keep to level ground for the first few weeks, then slowly introduce gentle hills, but avoid steep inclines.

Swimming This is a particularly beneficial exercise for arthritis, because it involves almost every muscle and joint in your body. The buoyancy of the water supports your weight; and exercising against the resistance of water increases strength, stamina, and suppleness. Even just walking through waist-high water is an excellent form of exercise. To get the most benefit from swimming, use a variety of different strokes and swim at least two or three times a week and preferably every day. Consider joining an aqua aerobics class

Exercise after joint replacement surgery

If you've had a hip or knee replacement, your orthopedic surgeon should advise you about which physical activities you can and can't do. When a group of surgeons working for the Mayo Clinic were asked which of several sports they would recommend to their patients following a hip or knee replacement, at least three-quarters agreed that the following activities were ideal: golf, swimming, cycling, sailing, scuba diving, and bowling. In addition, they recommended cross-country skiing after a knee replacement. Activities they would not recommend following either a hip or knee replacement included: squash, hockey, handball, baseball, running, water skiing, karate, basketball, soccer, football, and rugby. So, in general, participation in no-impact or low-impact sports is encouraged, but you should avoid taking part in high-impact sports.

at your local pool. Find out whether there are any hydrotherapy pools in your area—the water is warmer than in standard pools. For safety, never swim alone in case you develop severe pain or spasm while you are in the water.

Gardening This is an excellent form of exercise that can keep you fit and active. If you're a keen gardener, the following tips will help reduce strain on your joints:

- Don't try to do too much at once—gradually increase the amount of time you spend outdoors.
- Vary your activities—don't spend more than 20 to 30 minutes on each job.
- Use long-handled tools as much as possible to minimize bending or stooping.
- Use a spade and fork that are the right size for you. When buying a tool, go through the motions of planting, raking, digging, and so on to make sure the tool fits your build.
- Take only spadefuls of soil that are easy to handle comfortably.
- Consider installing raised beds and containers so you don't have to stoop.
- If you need to be near or on the ground, use a kneeling pad or low stool.
- Don't reach above shoulder level—always use a ladder.
- Load your wheelbarrow so the weight is mainly over the wheel, and bend your knees, not your back, to lift and lower the barrow.
- When you notice it's difficult to straighten up, stop.
- Whenever possible, get someone else to do the heavy work for you.

Warming up

Whatever form of exercise you do, warming up beforehand is vital to help unlock tight muscles and

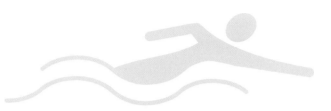

loosen stiff joints. Increasing your body temperature slightly boosts blood-flow to your muscles in preparation for extra exertion, and reduces the risk of cramp, tearing a muscle or spraining a ligament. Warming up also gets you into the right frame of mind.

Start with several deep breaths, inhaling through your nose and exhaling through your mouth. Then spend three to five minutes doing gentle exercises that use the muscles you will need for your exercise. One of the best warming-up exercises is to march on the spot, starting slowly and gradually speeding up. Then start to swing your arms at the same time, at a slow and gentle rate. Now add in some gentle stretches, such as a leg stretch (see page 97), hip stretch (see page 96), hamstring stretch (see page 155), shoulder stretch (see page 90), and arm stretch (see page 87).

Cooling down

Cooling down after exercise helps your muscles and joints relax. The cool-down routine is essentially the reverse of your warm-up routine, but, as your muscles are still warm and more elastic from your exercise, your muscles gain more benefit from the gentle stretches. Start with the stretches you performed in the warm-up, then finish with light aerobic exercise, such as walking, gently marching, or jogging on the spot. Cooling down reduces muscle fatigue and soreness, and keeps aches and pains to a minimum later. Both warming up and cooling down enhance flexibility, minimize discomfort, and prevent injury.

maintaining a healthy weight

Weight loss is one of the most effective ways to reduce pain in your knees and hips, whatever form of arthritis you have. It will also reduce your risk of other health problems, such as high blood pressure, raised cholesterol, coronary heart disease, stroke, and, possibly, some cancers.

When you walk, the load on your knees increases by four times your body weight. This means if you are 10 pounds overweight, the load on your leg joints is up to 40 pounds more than if you were at a healthy weight. If you are 28 pounds overweight, the load on your lower joints is 112 pounds greater than necessary with every step. And that's if you are walking on level ground. When walking downhill, the compressive force on your knees reaches eight times your body weight. This greatly increases the strain on your joints.

But, conversely, if you can lose just one pound in weight, there is at least a four-pound reduction in knee-joint load, which works out at around 4,800 pounds per one mil) walked.

The Arthritis Diet and Activity Promotion Trial (ADAPT) confirmed the effectiveness of moderate weight loss achieved through a combination of diet and exercise as a treatment for knee osteoarthritis. Those who combined modest weight loss with moderate exercise enjoyed a 24 percent improvement in their ability to perform daily activities, a reduction in morning stiffness, and significant improvements in mobility as well, as increase pain relief. Research shows weight loss can at least halve the level of pain experienced by people with arthritis affecting their lower limbs— that is a better result than standard drug treatments can achieve.

Losing weight

Use the chart on the opposite page to assess whether or not you need to lose any weight. Find your weight in pounds on the sides of the chart, and draw a line across at that level. Then, find your height in feet at the top or bottom of the graph, and draw a line up and down the chart. The point where these lines meet shows whether you are in the underweight, healthy, overweight, fat, or very fat range for your height.

If you're inactive as a result of joint pain, losing weight can be difficult, but not impossible. If you want to lose weight rapidly in the shortest possible time (for the quickest reduction in joint pain), I recommend a very low calorie diet (VLCD) with supervision. This provides less than 800 calories a day. VLCDs typically involve nutritionally complete vitamin and mineral-enriched drinks and meal replacement products. You can lose an average of 29–51 pounds excess weight within a year.

If you don't want to use meal replacement products and you're happy to lose weight over a longer period of time, I recommend a low-glycemic-index diet as your best weight-loss option. This restricts your intake of processed carbohydrates (which affect blood glucose levels, increase insulin secretion, and promote fat storage), while still providing the slowly digested carbohydrates in many fruits and vegetables. You can lose about 20 pounds after six months, on a low-glycemic diet. Many GI diet books are available to help guide you.

All of my diet plans in Part Three will also help you to lose some weight, although I haven't designed them as weight-loss programs. The healthy, low-glycemic eating plans should help you to shed weight slowly and naturally. Doing more exercise will also help you lose weight because it increases your metabolic rate and helps you burn more excess fat as a muscle fuel.

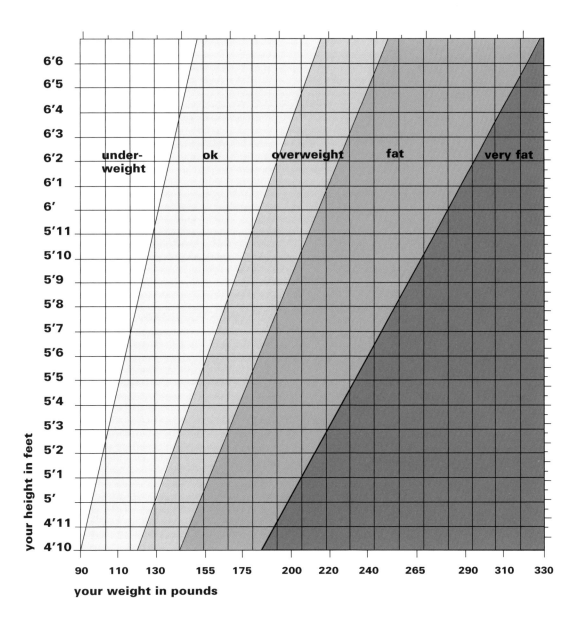

6'6
6'5
6'4
6'3
6'2   under-   ok   overweight   fat   very fat
6'1   weight
6'
5'11
5'10
5'9
5'8
5'7
5'6
5'5
5'4
5'3
5'2
5'1
5'
4'11
4'10

your height in feet

90 110 130 155 175 200 220 240 265 290 310 330

your weight in pounds

The natural health guru programs Having explained arthritis and the natural approaches to treating it in Parts One and Two, this section of the book provides you with three programs that offer **daily practical techniques to overcome arthritis**. First, I'd like you to complete a questionnaire that will help to pinpoint the best approach for you: the gentle, moderate, or full-strength program. **The gentle program** is aimed at people with a fair amount of dietary and lifestyle issues to address. It points you in the right direction with a healthy-eating, anti-inflammatory diet that's based around familiar, cosmopolitan dishes. **The moderate program** is designed for people whose arthritis symptoms are worsened by the chemicals found in foods from the nightshade family of plants (for example, tomatoes, potatoes, and bell peppers). Finally, **the full-strength program** provides an exceptionally high intake of natural antioxidants and anti-inflammatory spices. As well as **daily menus**, each program provides a nutritional **supplement plan**, recipes, an exercise routine, and **complementary therapies** to try. Each 14-day program is repeated once so the program lasts 28 days in total. Following one or more of the programs in Part Three should produce **significant improvements in your arthritis symptoms**.

the natural health guru questionnaire

There are three programs in this section of the book: the gentle, moderate, and full-strength programs. There are two ways to approach them: you can do each program sequentially, or you can start with the program that seems to best suit your needs.

Work through the programs in sequence

If you choose to do the programs one by one, the gentle program should be your starting point—this is an antioxidant-rich diet of fruit and vegetables, fish oils, anti-inflammatory spices, and other arthritis superfoods. After following the gentle program for a total of one month, you should notice a beneficial effect on your symptoms, in which case it's fine to stay on this program indefinitely. If not, it's possible that your arthritis symptoms are aggravated by the glycoalkaloids present in tomatoes, eggplants, potatoes, and chilies (see page 51). I'd therefore like you to move onto the moderate program, which is designed to eliminate these from your diet. If you *are* sensitive to these natural chemicals, a month of the moderate program should produce a marked improvement in your symptoms. If it doesn't, you can move onto the full-strength program. This provides an exceptionally high intake of anti-inflammatory antioxidants, plus a number of analgesic spices. If, after following the full-strength program for four weeks, your arthritis symptoms are still not significantly improved, you might have an idiosyncratic intolerance to some other component of your food intake. On page 50, I explain how to exclude the more common culprits from your diet, then reintroduce them one by one to identify any that appear to trigger your symptoms. You might also want to consult a naturopath or nutritional therapist who specializes in elimination diets to identify the foods to which you are sensitive.

Select the program that's best for you

If you already know or suspect that you're sensitive to the glycoalkaloids present in tomatoes, eggplants, potatoes, and chilies, it makes sense to start on the moderate program straight away. Alternatively, if you have severe pain and swelling, you'll need as many antioxidants as possible in your diet and I would advise starting on the full-strength program. I have also devised the questions on the next two pages to guide you toward the program that's best suited to your needs. When you've completed the questionnaire, work out which response you gave most frequently: A, B, or C; and, also, how many Bs or Cs you checked.

- If you answered mostly As: start with the gentle program—this is a gentle introduction to a therapeutic diet and it also gets you exercising.
- If you got five or more Bs, start on the moderate program. This excludes plants belonging to the nightshade family; some of your answers suggest these might make your arthritis symptoms worse.
- If you got five or more Cs, start on the full-strength program; your answers suggest that you're prepared for or in need of a high-antioxidant diet and an advanced routine of physical stretches.

1 Does arthritis run in your family?

- Don't know — A
- No — A/C
- Yes — C

2 Are your arthritis symptoms worse after eating chilies?

- Don't know — A/B
- Yes — B
- No — A/C

3 How many of your joints are affected by arthritis?

- One or two — A
- Three or four — A/C
- Five or more — C

4 Are your arthritis symptoms worse after eating eggplants?

- Don't know — A/B
- Yes — B
- No — A/C

5 How much pain have you had from your arthritis in the past week?

- Mild — A
- Moderate — A/C
- Severe — C

6 Are your joints very swollen?

- No — A
- A little — A/C
- Yes — C

7 Are your joints very inflamed?

- No — A
- A little — A/C
- Yes — C

8 Do you regularly feel lacking in energy or exhausted?

- Yes, most days — A
- Yes, most weeks — A
- No, not at all — C

9 Are your joints very stiff?

- No — A
- A little — A/C
- Yes — C

10 How often do you eat processed or prepackaged foods?

- Several times a day — A
- Several times a week — A/C
- Hardly ever — C

11 Do you take regular exercise?

- No — A
- Yes, I walk for 10 minutes three or four times a week — A/C
- Yes, for at least 20 minutes most days — C

12 How often do you eat carry-outs?

- Most days — A
- Several times a week — A/C
- Hardly ever — C

13 How often do you eat fried foods?

- Most days — A
- Several times a week — A/C
- Hardly ever — C

14 How many servings of fruit do you usually eat a day?

- One or less — A
- Two — A/C
- Three or more — C

15 Are your arthritis symptoms worse after eating tomatoes?

- Don't know — A/B
- Yes — B
- No — A/C

16 How many servings of vegetables or saladstuff do you usually eat a day?

- One or less — A
- Two — A/C
- Three or more — C

17 How often do you eat fish?

- Hardly ever — A
- Once or twice a week — A/C
- Three or more times a week — C

18 Are you willing to significantly change the way you eat?

- I'll start gently and see how I go — A
- Yes, but without going wild — A/B
- Yes, whatever it takes — B/C

19 Are your arthritis symptoms worse after eating bell peppers?

- Don't know — A/B
- Yes — B
- No — A/C

20 Can you pick up something from the floor?

- Don't know — A
- No — A
- Yes — C

21 Are your arthritis symptoms worse after eating potatoes?

- Don't know — A/B
- Yes — B
- No — A/C

22 Are your symptoms worse after exercise?

- Don't know — A
- No — A/C
- Yes — A

23 Can you reach up to get a heavy object?

- Don't know — A
- No — A
- Yes — C

24 Do you enjoy hot, spicy food?

- As long as it's not too hot — A
- No — A/B
- The hotter the better — C

25 Are you an adventurous eater?

- No, not at all — A
- I try to eat one new dish every week — A/C
- Yes, definitely — C

starting the programs

Once you've decided which program you're starting on, read through each day and make a list of the foods, supplements, and any other items you need to purchase—for example, magnetic jewelry (see page 96) or a crystal (see page 128). Book appointments with the appropriate complementary therapists, too. (See days seven and fourteen of each program.)

Whichever program you follow, it's important to monitor your progress. This will give you a clear indication of whether your arthritis symptoms are abating. Make a copy of the following chart and fill it in on the first day of a program and then at seven-day intervals. This chart will also be useful for your doctor to look at when reviewing your medication.

To complete the chart you'll need to assess the severity of your arthritis symptoms using a simple 0 to 10 scoring system. A score of 0 means you have no symptoms, 1 signifies very mild symptoms, 5 means moderate, and 10 means the most severe symptoms. It's also useful to include the number of painkillers, such as paracetamol or ibuprofen, you need to take each day, and your weight.

Progress chart for the gentle, moderate, and full-strength programs

	Day 1 of program	Day 7	Day 14	Day 21	Day 28
Date:					
Level of joint swelling (0–10):					
Level of joint stiffness (0–10):					
Level of muscle pain (0–10):					
Level of joint pain (0-10):					
Level of disability (0–10):					
Level of fatigue (0–10):					
Number of painkillers you need a day:					
Weight:					

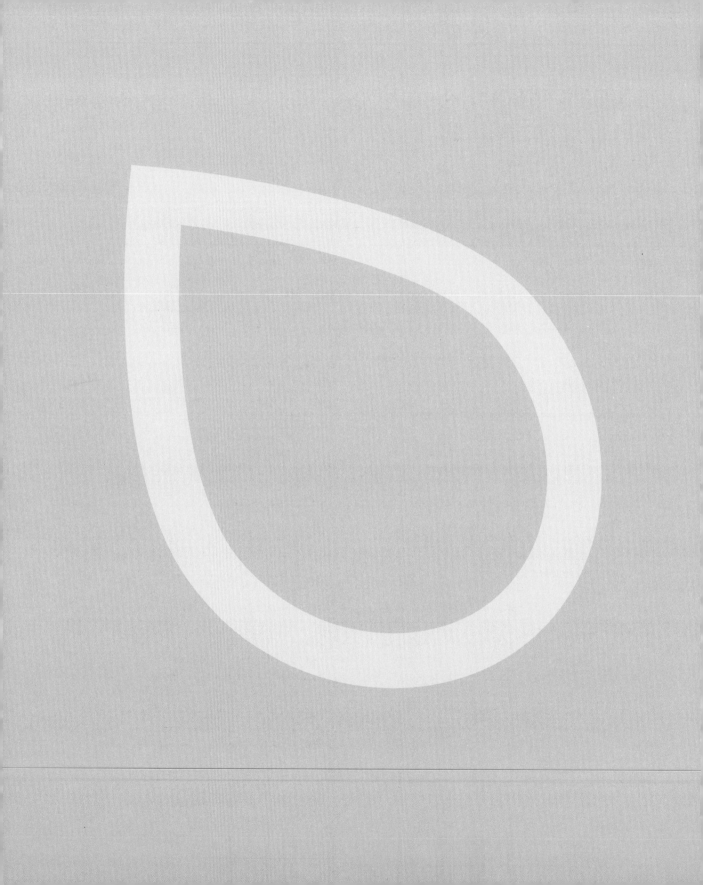

introducing the gentle program

My aim in the gentle program is to ease you into an arthritis-friendly diet and lifestyle that's simple to follow, yet effective at alleviating joint symptoms. It might take a while to settle into the program, but I'd like you to follow it for at least a month to obtain the full benefits. The program provides 14 daily plans you can repeat so it lasts for 28 days altogether. Once you get a feel for the diet and lifestyle changes involved, you can select your own changes to suit your personal likes and dislikes.

The gentle program diet

The diet you'll be following is an omega-3 enriched, anti-inflammatory diet that contains more fish, nuts, seeds, fruit, vegetables, salads, and wholegrains than you're probably used to. Olive oil and garlic also play a prominent role. This is a Mediterranean-style diet that is beneficial for "oiling" your joints and reducing pain, swelling, and stiffness. It's beneficial for people with all types of arthritis, and can produce significant reductions in pain when followed long term. It's even helpful for people with rheumatoid arthritis, as it decreases disease activity and reduces the risk of heart attack and stroke, to which people with rheumatoid arthritis are known to have an increased susceptibility (see page 13). As a bonus, the Mediterranean way to eat is good for both your immune function and mood regulation.

In addition to Mediterranean flavorings, such as garlic, I also include "gentle" spices, such as ginger, for their natural analgesic action.

You can read more about the arthritis superfoods I include in the gentle program on pages 54–57. You might be pleased to know bittersweet chocolate (choose products that contain at least 70 percent cocoa solids) and a couple of glasses of red wine a week are acceptable treats. Avoid these if they upset your arthritis symptoms, though.

Foods to avoid or eat less of I recommend you restrict your red meat intake to just two or three times a week—instead of meat for dinner I have included vegetarian or fish dishes on the majority of days. I have excluded added salt, convenience meals, and prepackaged snacks from the gentle program. Convenience and prepackaged foods, such as ready-to-heat meals, cakes, cookies, doughnuts, and pastries, contain omega-6 vegetable fats that promote inflammation in the body. Avoiding these foods can significantly help arthritis by increasing your antioxidant consumption and reducing the ratio of your intake of omega-6 oils compared with omega-3s.

Everyone with arthritis is different, and you might find that certain foods I have included in the gentle program seem to worsen your symptoms. If you notice a correlation between your symptoms and eating a particular food, make a point of eliminating that food (be aware of the impact of acid-forming foods; see pages 52–53). If you find that foods from the nightshade family upset your arthritis (tomatoes, potatoes, eggplants, bell peppers, and chilies; see page 51), follow the moderate program instead.

Shopping list

These are the items that feature in my suggested menu plans for the next 14 days. When possible, buy produce regularly for optimum freshness.

drinks
apple juice (unsweetened); fruit teas; tea (green, black, or white), ginger wine, herbal teas (ginger and rosehip), mineral water (low sodium), orange juice (freshly squeezed), wine (red and dry white)

dairy products
butter (unsalted), cheese (cheddar, feta, lowfat goat, Gruyère, mascarpone, mozzarella, Parmesan, and pecorino), ice cream (lowfat) milk (lowfat or nonfat), yogurt (lowfat with live cultures)

fruit
apples (eating and cooking), apricots (fresh and dried), bananas, blueberries, cranberries, figs, grapefruit (pink; see caution on page 83), grapes (black, red, green), kiwifruit, lemons, limes, melon, oranges, peaches, pears, pineapple, plums, pomegranate, raspberries, strawberries, tomatoes

vegetables
arugula, avocados, bean sprouts, beets, bell peppers (red and green), broccoli, butternut squash, carrots, corn, cucumber, eggplants, mixed salad leaves, mushrooms (cremini, mixed wild), onions (red and yellow), parsnips, peas, potatoes, romaine lettuce, rutabaga, scallions, spinach, spring greens, sweet potatoes, watercress, zucchini

nuts and seeds
almonds, Brazils, flax seeds (linseeds), macadamias, pecans, pine nuts, poppy seeds, pumpkin seeds, sesame seeds, sunflower seeds, walnuts

herbs, spices, oils, and vinegar
balsamic vinegar, basil, black pepper, bay leaves, chilies (fresh red and green), cilantro, cinnamon (ground and sticks), coriander seeds, cumin, garlic, ginger (ground and fresh), lemongrass, mustard seed, mint, nutmeg, olive oil (standard and extra virgin), oregano, parsley, red wine vinegar, rosemary, star anise, thyme, turmeric, vanilla (beans and extract), walnut oil

grains
bread (ciabatta, garlic bread, pita, and wholewheat bread and rolls), breakfast cereals (high-fiber wheatgerm and wholewheat cereals; instant oatmeal), flour (all-purpose and wholewheat), noodles, pasta (for example, fettuccine, spaghetti, and tagliatelle), quinoa, rice (brown)

proteins
eggs (omega-3-enriched), fish (cod, halibut, tuna—fresh and canned in olive oil—jumbo shrimp, salmon, and sardines), meat (chicken, lamb tenderloin, lean beef steaks, lean smoked bacon)

miscellaneous
almond nut milk, unsweetened cocoa powder, coconut cream, curry paste, bittersweet chocolate (at least 70 percent cocoa solids), phyllo pastry dough, fish sauce, honey, mayonnaise (lowfat), olive-oil spread, olives, pesto sauce, soy sauce, sugar (dark brown, Demerara, and superfine), tomato paste, vegetable bouillon cubes or stock

Drinking plenty of fluid Please drink plenty of fluids to help hydrate your joints—especially mineral water that contains good amounts of calcium and magnesium. Keep a small bottle of water with you at all times and take sips regularly throughout the day. Remember that by the time you feel thirsty, you are already significantly dehydrated. Herbal teas, such as ginger and rosehip, are also beneficial, as are antioxidant-rich black, green, and white teas.

Losing weight Although I haven't designed the gentle program as a weight-loss diet, you should find you lose any excess weight slowly and naturally. This is because you're likely to be eating fewer refined carbohydrates and saturated fats than you do normally. Both these contribute to excess fat, which can worsen arthritis in weight-bearing joints (see page 70). If you need to lose weight, you might want to enhance the process by eating smaller portions than I suggest in the gentle program and by cutting out some of the starchy foods suggested in each daily plan, such as the wholewheat toast and rolls.

The gentle program exercise routine

If you haven't exercised much in recent years, it's important to ease into a regular exercise program slowly to avoid aches and pains that might otherwise put you off. I'm going to give you a series of stretch exercises to perform, ideally twice a day, morning and evening. In addition, you should aim to do brisk aerobic exercise at least 15 minutes per day.

Walking is one of the easiest and cheapest ways to do aerobic exercise and increase your fitness level. You don't need any special skills or equipment and you can start immediately. I suggest that you buy a small pedometer to clip onto your clothes—this measures the number of steps you take in a day. The optimal number of paces per day for health is 10,000, but this

Gentle program supplements

These are the supplements that I feel are important to take on the gentle program. Take the ones in the recommended list and consider taking some or all of those on the optional list for even more benefits – read pages 58–63 to help you decide. Supplements are widely available in pharmacies, supermarkets and healthfood stores.

recommended daily supplements

- Vitamin C (500mg)
- Glucosamine sulphate (1500mg)
- Omega-3 fish oils (1g fish oil capsules, supplying 180mg EPA + 120mg DHA)
- Evening primrose oil (500mg)

optional daily supplements (these provide additional benefits)

- Vitamin-B complex (25mg)
- Vitamin D (5mcg)
- Vitamin E (200iu/134mg)
- Calcium (500mg)
- Selenium (50mcg)
- Green-lipped mussel extracts (200mg)

can present a significant challenge when your joints are stiff and painful. I suggest you build up slowly. Start by wearing a pedometer for a few days and simply record the number of steps you take in a day. Don't exert yourself or attempt to increase your level of activity dramatically. Round up the average number of steps you take to the nearest 1,000, then gradually try to increase this by 10 percent. So, for example, if you take 1,000 steps a day, aim to take 1,100 a day over the following week.

Once you are comfortable with a 10 percent increase, make an additional 10 percent increase. Keep building up your activity in these gradual stages over the course of your month on the gentle program. As well as increasing the number of steps you take, you can increase the speed at which you walk. Stop, however, if you feel you have reached your limit. Here is my suggested walking plan for the gentle program. This provides a structure within which you can build up your number of daily steps.

- Weeks one and two: walk 10 minutes a day on Tuesday, Thursday, and Saturday.
- Week three: walk 10 minutes a day on Tuesday and Saturday; and 15 minutes a day on Thursday and Sunday.
- Weeks four and onward: walk 15 minutes a day on Tuesday, Thursday, Saturday, and Sunday.

The gentle program therapies

My aim is to introduce you to some easy-to-follow techniques from some of the less-invasive holistic approaches. A number of complementary therapies can help to reduce the pain, swelling, and stiffness of arthritis. You can practice some, such as aromatherapy, acupressure, magnetic therapy, and meditation, as self-help techniques at home, while others are practitioner-led, at least initially. Before you begin the program I suggest that you book an appointment for an aromatherapy massage on day seven of the program, and with a homeopath on day fourteen.

the gentle program day one

Daily menu

- **Breakfast: Almond Oatmeal with Fresh Berries (see page 100)**

- **Morning snack: an apple**

- **Lunch: bowl of mixed salad leaves with Lemon and Olive Oil Dressing (see the box on page 96) sprinkled with feta cheese, olives, chopped tomatoes, red onions, and cucumber. Wholewheat pita bread. Lowfat yogurt with live cultures with fresh fruit**

- **Afternoon snack: a handful of walnuts**

- **Dinner: Cod in Soy Sauce (see page 106). Spinach. Mashed sweet potato. Corn. Figs in Red Wine (see page 108)**

- **Drinks: 2½ cups lowfat or nonfat milk. Unlimited tea (including herbal or fruit tea) and mineral water**

- **Supplements: see page 81**

I have included apple in every eating plan of the gentle program —either as a midmorning snack, or as part of your breakfast or dessert menus. Apples are a rich dietary source of anti-inflammatory antioxidants and, as I described on page 54, a fantastic superfood for arthritis.

Daily exercise routine

The stretch exercises I show you over the following two weeks will help improve your joint mobility, and strengthen your muscles and bones. Repeat them once or twice a day, adding each day's exercise onto the previous one so you build up a gentle stretch sequence. Start today with a neck stretch.

You might also like to start your walking routine, as outlined on pages 80–81. Walk for at least 10 minutes, three times a week during the first two weeks of the program. If you are already accustomed to walking regularly, then walk for 30 minutes, at least three times per week—and ideally every day. Remember to warm up and cool down (see page 89).

Neck stretch

1 Stand comfortably with your feet a little way apart and your shoulders relaxed.

2 Slowly drop your head so your left ear moves toward your left shoulder. Hold the stretch for a count of five. Now repeat on the right-hand side.

Aromatherapy

Tonight, I'd like you to place a few drops of lavender essential oil on a tissue or handkerchief and tuck it under your pillow when you go to bed to help you sleep.

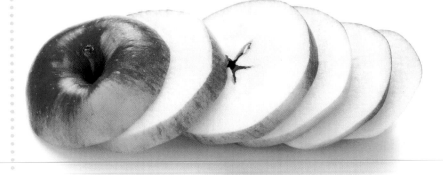

day two

Daily menu

- **Breakfast: bowl of high-fiber cereal. Pink grapefruit (see caution box on the right) sprinkled with ground ginger**

- **Morning snack: an apple**

- **Lunch: Avocado, Mozzarella, and Pepper Salad (see page 102). Wholewheat roll. Lowfat yogurt with live cultures with fresh fruit**

- **Afternoon snack: a handful of macadamia nuts**

- **Dinner: Mildly Spiced Broiled Chicken (see page 106). Broccoli. Carrots. Brown rice (cook extra for tomorrow's lunch). Strawberries in Balsamic Vinegar with Vanilla Mascarpone (see page 109)**

- **Drinks: 2½ cups lowfat or nonfat milk. Unlimited tea (including herbal or fruit tea) and mineral water**

- **Supplements: see page 81**

Daily exercise routine

Continue your walking routine, as outlined on pages 80–81. Remember to warm up and cool down. Do yesterday's neck stretch, then add the following shoulder stretch.

Shoulder stretch 1

1 Close your eyes and visualize yourself carrying a heavy briefcase in each hand —let your shoulders be pulled toward the floor.

2 Now imagine dropping the briefcases suddenly. Feel the weight and tension disappear and your shoulders and neck relaxing—your shoulders should move up a little as you do this. Repeat this five times.

Aromatherapy

Today, I'd like you to select a single essential oil from those suggested on page 27 (or you can continue to use lavender, or buy a massage oil or lotion). Add two drops of your chosen oil to 1 teaspoon carrier oil and massage into your hands. Rub vigorously to get your hand joints moving.

Grapefruit —check for interactions

Today's menu includes grapefruit. If you're taking any medications, check your drug information leaflet(s) for potential interactions with grapefruit. The antioxidant bioflavonoids present in grapefruit are beneficial for arthritis, but they can also increase absorption of some drugs. If your drug-insert sheet(s) says you should avoid grapefruit, replace the fruit with an orange —particularly a ruby or blood orange.

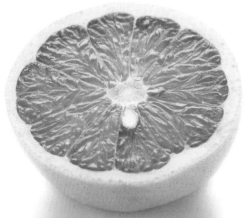

the gentle program day three

Daily menu

- **Breakfast: Apple, Pineapple, and Blueberry Smoothie (see page 100). Wholewheat toast with a scraping of olive-oil spread and honey**

- **Morning snack: a banana**

- **Lunch: Coronation Chicken (see instructions on the right). Bowl of brown rice mixed with chopped red bell pepper and parsley, and drizzled with Lemon and Olive Oil Dressing (see the box on page 96). Lowfat yogurt with live cultures with fresh fruit**

- **Afternoon snack: a handful of walnuts**

- **Dinner: Vegetable Gratinée with Basil and Walnuts (see page 107). Bowl of mixed salad leaves drizzled with olive oil. Crusty garlic bread. A handful of red grapes**

- **Drinks: 2½ cups lowfat or nonfat milk. Unlimited green, black, or white tea, herbal tea, and mineral water**

- **Supplements: see page 81**

Today's lunch is Coronation Chicken. To make it, mix together a handful of chopped fresh apricots with some cooked, shredded chicken breast, a dollop of lowfat mayonnaise, and 2 to 3 teaspoons curry paste, (you can add more than this—or less—depending on how spicy you like your food). Serve the chicken on a bed of lettuce.

Daily exercise routine

Continue your walking routine, as outlined on pages 80–81. Remember to warm up and cool down. Do the neck and shoulder exercises from the previous two days of the program, then add the following shoulder stretch to the sequence.

Shoulder stretch 2

1 Pretend that you're going to put your hands in the back pockets of your slacks—your aim is to move your shoulder blades together and bring your elbows as close together behind your back as you can manage.

2 Relax then repeat five times.

Aromatherapy

After massaging your hands as you did yesterday, use your essential oil blend (or a commerical massage lotion) to massage any painful joints in your feet as vigorously as you comfortably can. This will warm the joints and stimulate circulation. Now gently move your toes and ankles through their normal range of motion.

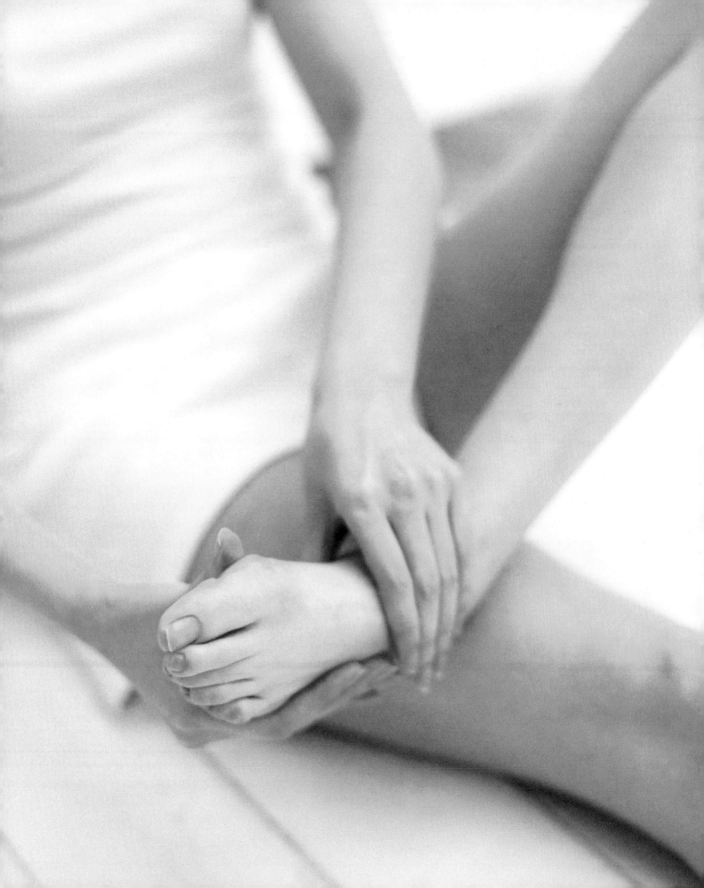

the gentle program day four

Daily menu

- **Breakfast: pink grapefruit (see the box on page 83) sprinkled with ground. Lowfat goat cheese on a slice of wholewheat bread, drizzled with walnut oil**

- **Morning snack: a pear**

- **Lunch: Chicken, Lime, and Grape Salad (see page 103). Wholewheat roll. Lowfat yogurt with live cultures with fresh fruit**

- **Afternoon snack: a handful of macadamia nuts**

- **Dinner: Thai Salmon-Phyllo Packages (see page 104). Sweet Chili Jelly (see page 104). Stir-fried bean sprouts and red bell peppers. Noodles. Plum, Apple, and Almond Crumble (see page 109)**

- **Drinks: 2½ cups lowfat or nonfat milk. Unlimited tea (including herbal or fruit tea) and mineral water**

- **Supplements: see page 81**

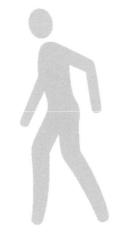

Daily exercise routine

Continue your walking routine, as outlined on pages 80–81. Remember to warm up and cool down. Do the stretch exercises from days one to three, then add the following arm stretch.

Arm stretch 1

1 Raise your arms above your head. Keep them straight and stretch as high as you can.
2 Lower your arms and let go of tension in your neck, shoulders, and arms. Repeat five times.

Aromatherapy

Massage your joints with an essential-oil blend or commercial massage lotion as on previous days of the program. Then soak your feet in the following essential-oil footbath. If you like, you can substitute your own favorite essential oils for the ones I suggest. If you find the footbath eases pain in your feet, or relaxes you generally, consider investing in a home-spa footbath.

Aromatherapy footbath

1 Add the following essential oils to a bowl of warm water: five drops of lavender, two drops of peppermint, and two drops of rosemary.
2 Sit in a comfortable chair with your feet resting in the water. Relax 15 minutes by reading a book or by closing your eyes and listening to your favorite piece of music.

Don't over-exert yourself
Perform your stretch exercises only if you can do so comfortably. If a stretch causes you discomfort, stop.

day five

Daily menu

- **Breakfast: Omega-3 Omelet with Tuna and Gruyère (see page 100). Slice of wholewheat bread with a scraping of olive-oil spread**

- **Morning snack: an apple**

- **Lunch: bowl of vegetable soup, such as, carrot and orange (see the box on page 93). Wholewheat roll. Lowfat yogurt with live cultures with fresh fruit**

- **Afternoon snack: a handful of walnuts**

- **Dinner: spaghetti with ragù sauce (use a bought sauce or make your own recipe). Mixed salad. Chocolate Cinnamon-Pecan Brownies (see page 108)**

- **Drinks: 2½ cups lowfat or nonfat milk. Unlimited tea (including herbal or fruit tea) and mineral water. Glass of red wine (optional)**

- **Supplements: see page 81**

Cutting back the amount of red meat you eat can relieve arthritis symptoms in some people (see pages 51–52). Today, I've included spaghetti with ragù sauce for dinner. (This will be your first exposure to red meat on the gentle program.) Please monitor your joint symptoms carefully over the next one to three days—if you notice they flare up, this might be a reaction to eating the red meat in the sauce. If this is the case for you, I recommend you avoid meat for the next two weeks. You will need to select a vegetarian meal option in place of the red meat on days eight, nine, and fourteen. After two weeks, try reintroducing meat to see if your arthritis flares up again. This elimination-and-challenge approach is an established way to identify the foods to which you might be intolerant (see page 50).

Daily exercise routine

Continue your walking routine (see pages 80–81). Remember to warm up and cool down. Do the stretch exercises from days one to four, then add in the following arm stretch.

Arm stretch 2

1 Interlink your fingers and turn your palms outward.
2 Extend your arms in front of you at shoulder height. Hold for 10 to 20 seconds. Relax, then repeat five times.

Heat treatment

Prepare some hot compresses as described on page 27. Place hot, wet cloths over your most painful joints. Let the compresses cool to body temperature, then remove; repeat two or three times. Then, gently move and stretch your joints to help improve their mobility.

the gentle program day six

Daily menu

- **Breakfast: Herbed Sardines on Toast (see page 101)**

- **Morning snack: an apple**

- **Lunch: bowl of chopped fresh pineapple, Brazil nuts, grated cheese, and mixed salad leaves, drizzled with Lemon and Olive oil Dressing (see the box on page 96). Wholewheat roll. Lowfat yogurt with live cultures with fresh fruit**

- **Afternoon snack: a handful of macadamia nuts**

- **Dinner: Mushroom and Walnut Roast (see page 107). Spring greens. Chunks of roasted butternut squash or sweet potato. Roast tomatoes. A handful of red grapes**

- **Drinks: 2½ cups lowfat or nonfat milk. Unlimited tea (including herbal or fruit tea) and mineral water**

- **Supplements: see page 81**

Sardines are an excellent source of omega-3 fatty acids. If you don't have time to make the herbed sardines on toast for today's breakfast, open a can of sardines or pilchards instead. Those canned in tomato sauce provide additional antioxidants in the form of lycopene—the red tomato carotenoid.

Daily exercise routine

Continue your walking routine, as described on pages 80–81. Make sure you warm up and cool down. Do the stretch exercises from days one to five, then add the following finger stretch.

Finger stretch

1 Sit down at a table and rest your hands on the tabletop with your palms facing down. Spread your fingers as wide as you can, and hold the stretch for a count of five.

2 Bring your fingers back together again, while keeping your palms flat on the table. Repeat both steps five times.

Aromatherapy

Today's therapeutic treatment is an analgesic aromatherapy bath.

1 Add three drops of lavender and two drops of rosemary essential oils to 1 tablespoon carrier oil.

2 Run your bath so it is comfortably hot, then add the aromatic oil mix after the faucet is turned off. Soak for 15 minutes, ideally in candlelight.

day seven

Daily menu

- **Breakfast: a punnet of wild mushrooms sautéed with garlic in a little olive oil. Wholewheat toast**

- **Morning snack: a banana**

- **Lunch: Quinoa, Apricot, Mozzarella, and Pomegranate Salad (see page 102). Lowfat yogurt with live cultures with fresh fruit**

- **Afternoon snack: a handful of walnuts**

- **Dinner: Braised Halibut with Sweet Peppers (see page 106). Broccoli. Corn. Baked potato. Mulled Cranberry Apples (see page 109)**

- **Drinks: 2½ cups lowfat or nonfat milk. Unlimited tea (including herbal or fruit tea) and mineral water**

- **Supplements: see page 81**

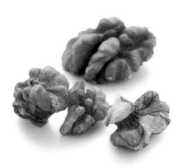

Warming up before aerobic exercise and cooling down afterward is important to maximize your joint flexibility and to prevent injury and discomfort. Use the stretching exercises in this program. When you go walking it helps to start at a slow speed; then, when your joints and muscles have warmed up, pick up your pace.

Daily exercise routine

Keep up the walking routine outlined on pages 80–81. Remember to warm up and cool down (see above). Do the stretch exercises from days one to six, then add this wrist stretch.

Wrist stretch

1 Rest your wrists and hands, palms facing down on a table in front of you. Bend both hands up toward you so you can feel a strong stretch in your wrists. Hold the stretch for a count of five.

2 Turn your hands over so they are resting palms upward. Now bend both hands up toward you again. Hold the stretch for a count of five before relaxing. Repeat each movement five times.

Consulting a therapist

Having followed the gentle program for one week, your joint symptoms should have started to improve. I now suggest you consolidate these gains by visiting an aromatherapist for a relaxing, yet therapeutic, aromatherapy massage. An aromatherapist will select essential oils that will help ease painful, stiff joints. A full-body massage lasts about 60 minutes and you should feel relaxed afterward. If you enjoy the massage and find that it helps relieve pain and stiffness, book yourself in for a session over each of the next four weeks. To find an aromatherapist, check the resources at the end of this book.

the gentle program day eight

Daily menu

- **Breakfast: Almond Oatmeal with Fresh Berries (see page 100)**

- **Morning snack: an apple**

- **Lunch: tuna and corn salad or sandwich. Bowl of mixed lettuce leaves drizzled with Lemon and Olive Oil dressing (see the box on page 96). Lowfat yogurt with live cultures with fresh fruit**

- **Afternoon snack: a handful of macadamia nuts**

- **Dinner: Herby Lamb and Eggplant Kabobs (see page 106). Brown rice. Bowl of mixed salad leaves drizzled with Lemon and Olive Oil Dressing (see the box on page 96). Figs in Red Wine (see page 108)**

- **Drinks: 2½ cups lowfat or nonfat milk. Unlimited tea (including herbal or fruit tea) and mineral water**

- **Supplements: see page 81**

Over the next few days I introduce you to to several different complementary therapies that are beneficial for arthritis. Everyone is different, with different likes and dislikes, so once you've found a therapy that suits you, find other ways to incorporate it into your treatment routine. The first complementary technique I'd like you to try is hand reflexology.

Daily exercise routine

Continue to walk three times a week (or more often if your joints allow you to), making sure you warm up and cool down. Do the stretch exercises from days one to seven, then add in the following shoulder stretch.

Shoulder stretch

1 Stand comfortably with your feet apart. Raise your arms and clasp your hands behind your head. Pull your elbows forward so they are as close together as possible in front of your face. Hold the stretch for a count of five.

2 Now gently swing your elbows out so they are as wide apart as possible. Hold the stretch for a count of five.

Hand reflexology

The underlying principle of reflexology is that parts of your body are represented by "reflexes" on your hands and feet, so massaging the appropriate reflex on your hands or feet can heal the linked body part. Look at the illustrations on pages 38 and 39 and identify the reflex on your hand that relates to your painful joint/s. Gently massage this area on each hand for two minutes. Do this whenever your joints ache.

Hugging therapy

Next time your joint pains start to get you down, indulge in some hugging therapy. Hugging or cuddling someone helps to decrease your perception of pain. This is because hugging triggers the release of oxytocin, a hormone involved in bonding that increases your pain threshold. Hugging a pet works just as well as hugging a human.

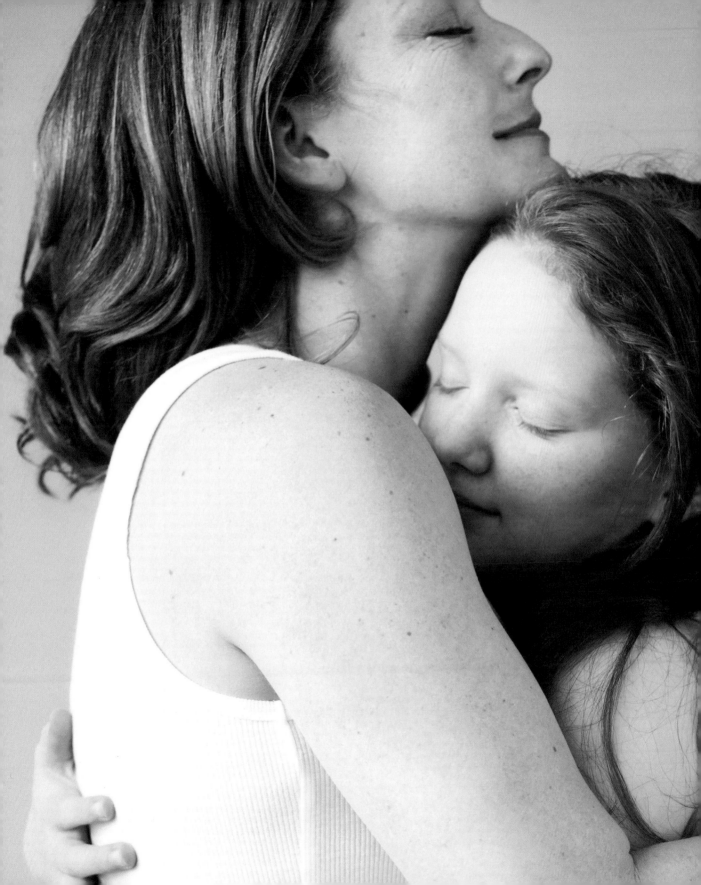

the gentle program day nine

Daily menu

- **Breakfast: plate of fresh fruit: for example, orange, kiwifruit, and grapes. Bowl of high-fibre cereal**

- **Morning snack: an apple**

- **Lunch: Avocado and Bacon Salad with Beet Mayonnaise (see page 102). Wholewheat roll. Yogurt with live cultures with fresh fruit**

- **Afternoon snack: a handful of walnuts**

- **Dinner: pasta in pesto sauce. Bowl of mixed salad leaves drizzled with Lemon and Olive Oil Dressing (see the box on page 96). Strawberries in Balsamic Vinegar with Vanilla Mascarpone (see page 109)**

- **Drinks: 2½ cups lowfat or nonfat milk. Unlimited tea (including herbal or fruit tea) and mineral water**

- **Supplements: see page 81**

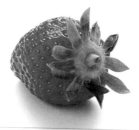

A high intake of fruit is important when you have arthritis. The antioxidants present in fruit help to reduce inflammation and slow the rate of cartilage breakdown in joints. Today's breakfast gives you a head start.

Daily exercise routine

Continue to walk at least three times a week (see pages 80–81). Remember to warm up and cool down. Do the stretch exercises from days one to eight, then add in the following torso stretch.

Torso stretch

1 Stand comfortably with your feet apart and your hands on your hips. Without moving your lower body, rotate your upper body and hips to the right as far as you can. Hold the stretch for a count of five.
2 Rotate back to the front and

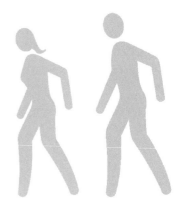

repeat toward the left. Repeat five times in each direction.

Acupressure

Today I recommend you try acupressure to help with your arthritis symptoms. Acupoints around a tender joint often become very sensitive. Press gently around a joint to find the most tender spot and press on it for 10 seconds; relax and repeat. Do the same on the other side. See the box on page 42 for more on acupressure.

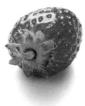

day ten

Daily menu

- Breakfast: slice of melon. Hard-boiled omega-3-enriched egg. Wholewheat toast with a scraping of olive-oil spread

- Morning snack: an apple

- Lunch: bowl of vegetable soup, such as tomato and basil (see the box on the right). Wholewheat roll. Lowfat yogurt with live cultures with fresh fruit

- Afternoon snack: a handful of macadamia nuts

- Dinner: Shrimp and Coconut Curry (see page 105). Brown or red rice. 1 to 1½ ounces bittersweet chocolate (at least 70 percent cocoa solids)

- Drinks: 2½ cups lowfat or nonfat milk. Unlimited tea (including herbal or fruit tea) and mineral water

- Supplements: see page 81

The arnica gel you are using today is prepared using the principles of homeopathy and, after immense dilution, contains no measurable amount of arnica. This is different from herbal arnica gel, which contains measurable amounts of the herb (typically from one to 25 percent of *Arnica montana* extract). Make sure you buy a homeopathic version of the gel for the gentle program.

A study involving 172 people with osteoarthritis of the knee compared the use of a homeopathic arnica gel with an NSAID (piroxicam) gel. Results showed the homeopathic gel was at least as effective and as well tolerated as the NSAID gel.

Homemade soup

It is easy to make a bowl of healthy vegetable soup by slowly simmering together chopped mixed vegetables, tomatoes, herbs, and sometimes fruit in water or stock. When cooked, puree the vegetables to make a thick, smooth soup, or leave them in chunks, if you prefer. Good combinations are tomato and basil, as in today's lunch; carrot and orange; carrot and cilantro; leek and potato; and parsnip and apple.

Daily exercise routine

Continue your walking routine as described on pages 80–81. Remember to warm up and cool down. Do the stretch exercises from days one to nine, then add the following ankle stretch.

Ankle stretch

1 Stand comfortably with your feet slightly apart and one hand resting on the back of a nearby chair or a table for support. Lift both heels up so you are standing on the balls of your feet.

2 Lower your heels down to the floor and relax. Do 10 to 15 complete movements.

Homeopathy

I'd like you to buy a homeopathic preparation of arnica gel to rub into your affected joints. Apply the gel two or three times a day for at least the next five days.

the gentle program day eleven

Daily menu

- **Breakfast: Mediterranean Sauté (see page 101)**
- **Morning snack: a pear**
- **Lunch: chicken salad or sandwich. Lowfat yogurt with live cultures with fresh fruit**
- **Afternoon snack: a handful of macadamia nuts**
- **Dinner: roast chicken. Roast sweet potato. Spinach. Carrots. Peas. Plum, Apple, and Almond Crumble (see page 109)**
- **Drinks: 2½ cups lowfat or nonfat milk. Unlimited tea (including herbal or fruit tea) and mineral water**
- **Supplements: see page 81**

Daily exercise routine

Keep up your three-times-a-week walking routine (see pages 80–81), walking farther or more frequently as soon as you feel able to. Remember to warm up and cool down. Do the stretch exercises from days one to ten, then do the following hip stretch.

Hip stretch 1

1 Stand comfortably with your feet slightly apart and one hand resting on a table for support. Raise your left knee with your leg bent. Bring it up as high in front of you as is comfortable. Feel the stretch in your left hip. Hold for a count of five.
2 Now do the same with the right knee. Repeat the stretch on both sides five times.

Herbalism

Today, I'd like you to start using a herbal medicine to help your arthritis symptoms. The one I've selected as most appropriate for the gentle program is bromelain, an anti-inflammatory extract from the stems of the pineapple plant (*Ananas comosus*). It can significantly reduce acute knee pain, and the stiffness and swelling associated with osteoarthritis and rheumatoid arthritis. It can also reduce pain and bruising after surgery. It is not suitable for everyone, however. You shouldn't take it if you're taking blood-thinning medication, such as aspirin, because bromelain also thins the blood. If you want to take it to minimize post-surgical pain and bruising, please check with your surgeon before doing so.

If you can take bromelain, start with a 300 mg supplement once or twice a day depending on the severity of your symptoms. If you can't take bromelain, consider taking another herb that will help your arthritis—see page 28 for suggestions.

day twelve

Daily menu

- **Breakfast: oatmeal swirled with applesauce**

- **Morning snack: a large apple**

- **Lunch: Chicken, Lime, and Grape Salad (see page 103). Wholegrain roll. Lowfat yogurt with live cultures with fresh fruit**

- **Afternoon snack: a handful of macadamia nuts**

- **Dinner: vegetarian stew, such as carrots, corn, rutabaga, tomatoes, squash, and zucchini simmered in vegetable stock with a handful of chopped fresh herbs. Crusty garlic bread. Chocolate Cinnamon-Pecan Brownies (see page 108)**

- **Drinks: 2½ cups lowfat or nonfat milk. Unlimited tea (including herbal or fruit tea) and mineral water. Glass of red wine (optional)**

- **Supplements: see page 81**

I have included an optional glass of red wine on days five and twelve of the gentle program. Red wine is a rich source of anti-inflammatory antioxidants, but it doesn't suit everyone. Some people with arthritis find that it triggers flare-ups of joint pain. If you notice your arthritis symptoms worsen over the next day or two, and the same thing happened after drinking red wine last week, it's advisable to abstain.

Daily exercise routine

Continue your walking routine, as outlined on pages 80–81. Remember to warm up and cool down. Do the stretch exercises from days one to eleven, then do the following hip stretch.

Hip stretch 2

1 Stand comfortably with your feet slightly apart and one hand on a table for support. Keep your left leg straight and move it out to the side of your body as far as feels comfortable. Hold for a count of five.

2 Now do the same with the right leg. Repeat on both sides five times.

Meditation

This is a simple meditation technique to help reduce joint pain.

Color meditation

1 Sit comfortably in a chair with your eyes shut. Picture a purple color (purple is healing) and leave it to swirl behind your eyelids. The more color you can visualize, the stronger the healing effect. If your mind wanders, keep returning to focus on the color purple.

2 When you feel ready, bring your mind slowly back, open your eyes, and enjoy the sense of calm that flows through you. Try to meditate for at least five minutes a day from now on, building up to 15 minutes or longer over time.

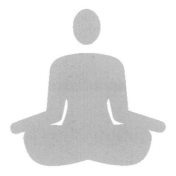

the gentle program
day thirteen

Daily menu

- **Breakfast: Herbed Sardines on Toast (see page 101)**

- **Morning snack: an apple**

- **Lunch: Butternut Squash and Rosemary Pasta (see page 103). Lowfat yogurt with live cultures with fresh fruit**

- **Afternoon snack: a handful of walnuts**

- **Dinner: Mildly Tikka Fish (see page 105). Brown rice. Bowl of mixed salad leaves drizzled with Lemon and Olive Oil Dressing (see the box on the right). A handful of red grapes**

- **Drinks: 2½ cups lowfat or nonfat milk. Unlimited tea (including herbal or fruit tea) and mineral water**

- **Supplements: see page 81**

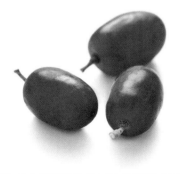

Today, I've suggested a cooked lunch of pasta with butternut squash and rosemary. It's quick and easy to make, but if you're short of time, cook fresh pasta in boiling water three minutes (or follow the package directions) and combine with bottled pesto sauce instead.

Daily exercise routine

Continue your walking routine (see pages 80–81). Remember to warm up and cool down. Do the stretch exercises from days one to twelve, then add the following hip stretch.

Hip stretch 3

1 Stand comfortably with your feet slightly apart. Put one hand on a table for support.
2 Bend your right knee and lift your right foot up behind you as far as feels comfortable—try to grasp your ankle with your right hand. Your knees should face forward: do not twist them.
3 If you've grasped your ankle, gently ease your foot in toward your right buttock until you feel a mild stretch. Hold for a count of five. Repeat the stretch on your left leg.

Magnetic jewelry

I'd like you to invest in a piece of magnetic jewelry or an accessory, such as a bracelet, belt, ring, watch, or necklace, to wear all the time from now on. Magnetic therapy improves circulation and promotes healing in the area where it's worn. In one study of the effects of magnets, magnetic patches were found to be 80-percent effective in relieving painful, stiff shoulders, whereas nonmagnetized placebos were only six-percent effective.

Lemon and olive oil dressing

Throughout the gentle program I've suggested a simple Lemon and Olive Oil Dressing to drizzle over your salad. Lemons are rich in vitamin C, and olive oil is an arthritis superfood (see page 56). To make the dressing simply shake 4 tablespoons extra virgin olive oil together with the grated zest and juice of one large unwaxed lemon. Season with plenty of freshly ground black pepper.

day fourteen

Daily menu

- **Breakfast: pink grapefruit sprinkled with ground ginger (see the caution on page 83). Bowl of high-fiber cereal**

- **Morning snack: a pear**

- **Lunch: French Onion Soup (sauté thinly sliced onions in a little olive oil until caramelized, then add some vegetable or meat stock, heat through, and season). Wholewheat roll. Lowfat yogurt with live cultures with fresh fruit**

- **Afternoon snack: a handful of macadamia nuts**

- **Dinner: small steak or chop, marinated in olive oil, garlic, and herbs, seasoned with black pepper, and broiled. Bowl of mixed salad leaves drizzled with Lemon and Olive Oil Dressing (see box on the left). Crusty garlic bread. Mulled Cranberry Apples (see page 109)**

- **Drinks: 2½ cups lowfat or nonfat milk. Unlimited tea (including herbal or fruit tea) and mineral water**

- **Supplements: see page 81**

Daily exercise routine

Continue the walking routine that I described on pages 80–81. From tomorrow start walking on four days a week instead of three (and increase the amount of time you walk by five minutes or more on two of the days). Always warm up before and cool down after your daily walk (or any other form of aerobic exercise). Do the stretch exercises from days one to thirteen, then add the following leg stretch.

Leg stretch

1 Lie on a comfortable surface, such as an exercise mat. Bend both knees so your feet are flat on the floor.

2 Lift one leg up in the air and straighten it. Hold for a count of five. Repeat with the other leg. When straightening one leg, always keep the other knee bent to protect your back. Don't try to lift both legs in the air at the same time.

Consulting a homeopath

Having followed the gentle program for two weeks, you should be experiencing less joint pain and stiffness, and greater mobility. I'd now like you to visit a homeopath. In one study, among 23 people with rheumatoid arthritis, homeopathy significantly improved subjective pain, stiffness and grip strength, while 23 similar people using a placebo did not show any significant benefit. A homeopath will choose a remedy specifically for you, based on your symptoms and constitutional type. Homeopaths recognize 15 different constitutional types, based on factors such as your build, personality, likes, dislikes, and emotions. Prescribing according to constitutional type is important when treating a long-term condition such as arthritis, for which there are many remedies. To find a homeopath, check the resources on page 175.

> **Mind your back!**
> Don't do today's exercise if it causes discomfort in your back or if you have back problems. Repeat yesterday's hip stretch instead.

continuing the gentle program

Congratulations—you have followed the gentle program for two weeks. Now I suggest you repeat the program one more time, so it lasts for 28 days in total. You can vary the foods you eat, and include some new recipes to introduce variety. You will find extra recipe suggestions at www.naturalhealthguru.co.uk and can post your own favorites there, too, for other followers of the program to try.

If you found the gentle program effective in relieving your symptoms and improving your general mobility and well-being, I advise you to stay on it long term. The following information helps you map out your future using the gentle program principles.

Your long-term diet

The menu plans in the gentle program form part of a healthy, anti-inflammatory diet that encourages consumption of wholegrain foods, fruit, vegetables, salads, lowfat dairy products, fish, nuts, and anti-inflammatory spices, such as ginger, chili, and turmeric. The diet also cuts back on your intake of red meat, sugar, saturated fats, and salt.

Continue to eat at least five (and preferably eight to 10) servings of fruit, vegetables, and salad ingredients a day, and aim for a wide range of colors on your plate —the colors in fruit and vegetables are a result of the variety of antioxidant pigments they contain. Check the information on pages 54–57 so you know which are the best superfoods to include in your diet when you have arthritis. Eat a handful of nuts per day, and select wholewheat bread, pasta, and cereals rather than processed white versions. Aim to eat two to four portions of fish—especially oily fish—a week if you can (see box below). If you don't like fish, or are unable to eat it, make sure you take omega-3 fish-oil supplements (see page 61), which are very important for joint health.

Eat red meat only occasionally and, then, have a relatively small serving of three ounces lean meat. Select omega-3-enriched hen eggs whenever possible, because, unlike standard hen eggs, these have beneficial effects on your blood cholesterol levels. Continue to avoid processed, packaged foods, which tend to contain high amounts of the omega-6 essential fatty acids that are converted into inflammatory substances in the body.

Oily fish

Oily fish is an important food in the gentle program diet. All of the following are categorized as oily fish: anchovies, bloater, cacha, carp, eel, herring, hilsa, jackfish, katla, kipper, mackerel, orange roughy, pangas, pilchards, salmon, sardines, sprats, swordfish, trout, tuna (fresh, not canned), and whitebait. Eat oily fish regularly, but note the advice given in some countries, such as the UK: girls and women who might become pregnant at some time should limit their intake to two portions a week. This is because sea pollutants, such as mercury, can affect the health of future offspring. Everyone else can eat oily fish up to four times a week.

Losing weight If you need to lose weight, cut back on the amount of carbohydrate you eat (for example, bread, rice, pasta, and couscous). Aim to eat only as much as you need to feel satisfied—don't feel you have to finish every item on your plate. You can always eat a bit more in an hour or two when you feel hungry again. In fact, having several small meals per day is more beneficial for weight loss than eating larger meals three times a day.

Avoiding trigger foods If you recognize that certain foods trigger a flare-up in your arthritis symptoms, cut them out of your diet, even if they are recognized arthritis superfoods. Everyone is different and your immune system might have developed an oversensitivity to certain foods. Consult a naturopath or a nutritionist with training in the field of food intolerances to help pinpoint the foods you react against. If you notice foods from the Solanaceae plant family (for example, tomatoes, potatoes, eggplants, and chilies) upset your joint symptoms, you might want to move onto the moderate program, which eliminates these foods.

Your long-term supplement regime

Continue taking the recommended supplements for the gentle program (see page 81) long term if they seem to be working for you. Research supports their use at this level for gentle, yet significant, effects on joint health. If your joint pain is not yet well controlled, and you are not currently taking all the supplements in the recommended list, you might want to add in those you have left out. Similarly if, up until now, you have only been taking only the supplements in the recommended list, you can add one or more of the supplements in the optional list. Read pages 58–63 to find out more about the supplements in which you are interested.

Your exercise routine

After two weeks of regular joint stretching exercises, you should have started to notice an increase in flexibility. Continue to do these stretch exercises, ideally twice a day. If you feel able to do more, try the stretch exercises in the moderate program.

You should also maintain your aerobic exercise routine. In the third week of the gentle program you should have started to walk four days a week instead of three (see page 80–81). If you're already walking more frequently and for longer than I suggest on page 81, that's great—just keep increasing the number of paces you take a day and stop when you feel you've reached a comfortable limit. If you want a change from walking, try other activities, such as cycling, swimming, dancing, gardening, bowling, and golf—try whatever activities you like doing and your joints allow you to do.

Your therapy program

The gentle program has shown you how to use aromatherapy and other techniques, such as magnetic therapy, homeopathy, herbal medicine, and meditation. If you found their treatments useful, continue to consult the natural healthcare professionals, such as the aromatherapist and homeopath I suggested you find on days seven and fourteen.

Monitoring your joint symptoms

While continuing on the gentle program I suggest you monitor and score your joint symptoms weekly. This enables you to see if you are continuing to benefit from the program. If your joint scores stop improving, or if they start to worsen again, I suggest you increase the level of supplements you take to that suggested for the moderate program (see page 113). You might also want to move onto the moderate program.

breakfast recipes

almond oatmeal with fresh berries

....

serves 4

2½ cups almond nut milk
Scant 2 cups old-fashioned rolled oats
¼ teaspoon ground cinnamon
1 handful slivered almonds
1 handful fresh berries

1 Bring the milk just to boiling point in a saucepan. Add the oats and cinnamon. Simmer gently 1 minute (or follow the directions on the package) while stirring.

2 Remove from the heat, cover, and leave to stand at least 5 minutes until all the liquid is absorbed. Sprinkle the almonds and berries on top and serve.

apple, pineapple, and blueberry smoothie

....

serves 4

2⅓ cups old-fashioned rolled oats
1 red eating apple, cored
1 pineapple, peeled, cored, and cut into chunks
1 handful blueberries
½ cup unsweetened apple juice

1 Put the ingredients in a food processor and blend until smooth. Add more or less apple juice if you prefer a lighter or thicker smoothie.

omega-3 omelet with tuna and gruyère

....

serves 4

8 omega-3-enriched eggs
2 tablespoons olive oil
1 handful grated Gruyère cheese
1 can (6½-oz.) flaked tuna in olive oil, drained
1 handful chopped parsley
Freshly ground black pepper

1 Beat the eggs lightly and season with plenty of black pepper.

2 Heat the olive oil in a large nonstick skillet over high heat. Tip in the eggs and gather the curds into the middle as the egg sets.

3 When there is only a little runny egg left, remove the pan from the heat. Scatter the Gruyère and tuna over one half of the omelet. Season with more black pepper.

4 Return to the heat and warm through 30 seconds. Flip the uncovered side of the omelet over. Slide out onto a plate, sprinkle with parsley, and serve.

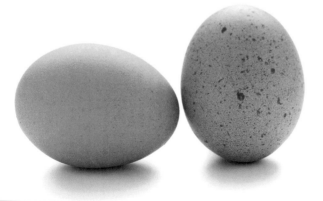

herbed sardines on toast

serves 4

4 fresh sardines, cleaned
2 tablespoons olive oil
1 small red onion, sliced
1 handful chopped herbs, such as
    oregano, thyme, rosemary, basil, and
    parsley
1 garlic clove, crushed
8 cherry tomatoes, halved
Grated zest and juice of ½ unwaxed
    lemon
4 slices wholewheat bread, toasted
Freshly ground black pepper

1 Brush the sardines with olive oil
   and sauté them with the onion,
   herbs, and garlic until they start
   to turn golden.
2 Add the tomatoes and lemon
   zest and juice and simmer
   slowly 5 minutes, or until
   cooked through.
3 Put the sardine mixture
   on the slices of toast,
   season well with black
   pepper, and serve.

mediterranean sauté

serves 4

4 tablespoons extra virgin olive oil
1 red onion, sliced
1 garlic clove, crushed
1 handful chopped herbs, such as
    oregano, thyme, rosemary, basil, and
    parsley
4 mushrooms, wiped and chopped
8 cherry tomatoes, halved
2 small zucchini, chopped
1 red bell pepper, seeded and cut
    into strips
1 green bell pepper, seeded and cut
    into strips
1 baby eggplant, chopped
4 slices wholewheat bread, toasted
Freshly ground black pepper

1 Heat the olive oil in a pan and
   sauté the red onion, garlic,
   and herbs 2 minutes. Add
   the remaining vegetables and
   sauté 5 minutes longer, or until
   cooked to your liking.
2 Put the vegetables on the
   slices of toast, season well
   with black pepper, and serve.

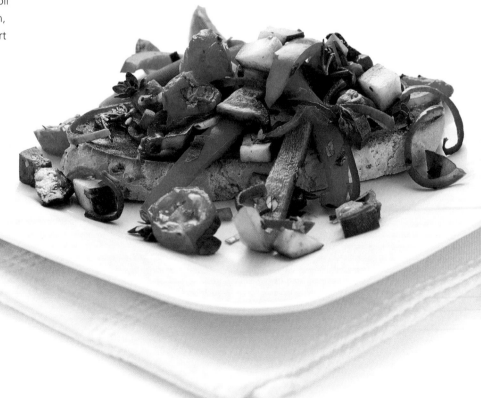

mediterranean sauté

lunch recipes

quinoa, apricot, mozzarella, and pomegranate salad

. . . .

serves 4

Heaped 1 cup quinoa
8 semidried apricots, chopped
1 handful mixed seeds and nuts, such
    as pumpkin, sesame, sunflower,
    poppy, flax seeds (linseeds), and
    pine nuts
1 pomegranate
2 buffalo mozzarella balls, drained and
    chopped
1 handful chopped cilantro leaves
4 handfuls mixed lettuce leaves
Freshly ground black pepper

1 Cook the quinoa according to
the package directions, then
drain and rinse it. Put it in the
refrigerator to chill.

2 Halve the pomegranate and,
holding each half over a large
bowl, bash the outer skin
with a wooden spoon until
all the seeds fall out into the
bowl. Mix together with the
chilled quinoa and all the other
remaining ingredients, except
the lettuce and pepper. Season
with black pepper, then put on
top of the lettuce and serve.

avocado and bacon salad with beet mayonnaise

. . . .

serves 4

6 slices lean, smoked bacon
2 avocados, peeled, pitted, and sliced
Grated zest and juice of 1 unwaxed
    lemon
12 cherry tomatoes, halved
4 scallions, chopped
½ cucumber, chopped
1 cup thinly sliced pecorino cheese
4 handfuls mixed baby salad leaves
Freshly ground black pepper

For the beet mayonnaise:
1 small beet, unpeeled
Scant ½ cup lowfat mayonnaise
1 tablespoon red wine vinegar

1 Broil the bacon until crispy.
Leave it to cool, then break it
into small pieces.

2 Mix the avocado with the
lemon zest and juice. Add the
remaining salad ingredients,
season well with black pepper,
and put in a bowl.

3 Boil the beet 30 minutes, or
until tender. Peel then blend
the beet with the mayonnaise
in a blender. Add the red wine
vinegar. Serve the salad with
the beet mayonnaise.

avocado, mozzarella, and pepper salad

. . . .

serves 4

2 avocados, peeled, pitted, and sliced
Grated zest and juice of 1 unwaxed
    lemon
1 red bell pepper, seeded and chopped
1 handful basil leaves, torm
4 ounces mini mozzarella balls, drained
1 handful walnuts, chopped
4 tablespoons walnut oil
1 ciabatta, sliced and toasted
Freshly ground black pepper

1 Mix the avocado slices with the
lemon zest and juice to prevent
discoloration. Add the red
bell pepper, basil, mozzarella,
walnuts, and walnut oil and
leave to infuse 30 minutes.

2 Put the salad on the ciabatta
slices, season with black
pepper, and serve.

chicken, lime, and grape salad

serves 4

4 boneless chicken breast halves
2 tablespoons olive oil
Grated zest and juice of 4 unwaxed limes
1 red onion, finely chopped
1 garlic clove, crushed
2 tablespoons fish sauce
1 tablespoon sugar
1 romaine lettuce, chopped
6 ounces red grapes
A few sprigs mint, chopped
Freshly ground black pepper

1 Heat the oven to 400°F. Brush the chicken with some of the olive oil and half the lime juice. Roast 20 minutes, or until cooked through.

2 Heat the remaining oil in a pan and sauté the onion and garlic until soft. Add the remaining lime zest and juice, fish sauce, and sugar.

3 Toss the lettuce leaves and grapes in the sauce. Put the chicken on top of the lettuce, pour the sauce over, season with black pepper, sprinkle with the mint, and serve.

butternut squash and rosemary pasta

serves 4

6 tablespoons unsalted butter
2 garlic cloves, crushed
3 cups peeled, seeded butternut squash, cut into bite-size pieces
5 sprigs rosemary, finely chopped
Grated zest and juice of 1 unwaxed lemon
1 pound fresh pasta or 12 ounces dried pasta
¼ teaspoon freshly ground nutmeg
½ cup freshly shaved Parmesan cheese
Freshly ground black pepper

1 Melt the butter in a pan and sauté the garlic 30 seconds. Add the squash, the chopped leaves of 1 rosemary sprig, and the lemon zest and juice. Cover and sweat over low heat 15 minutes, stirring occasionally.

2 Meanwhile, cook the pasta according to the package directions, then drain.

3 Mash half the squash into the butter. Season with black pepper and nutmeg. Mix the pasta with the squash, sprinkle the remaining rosemary and Parmesan on top, and serve.

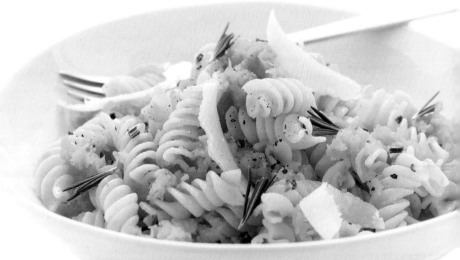

butternut squash and rosemary pasta

dinner recipes

thai salmon-phyllo packages

• • • • • • • • • • • • • • • • • • • •

serves 4

4 salmon fillet steaks
4 sheets phyllo pastry dough
4 tablespoons Sweet Chili Jelly (see
    following recipe)
4 tablespoons butter, melted

1 Heat the oven to 400°F. Put
    a fillet of salmon at the end
    of each piece of phyllo pastry
    dough. Use some of the Sweet
    Chili Jelly to coat the fish.

2 Brush the surrounding dough
    with some of the melted
    butter and wrap up the salmon,
    folding the sides in to make
    a neat package. Repeat with
    the remaining pieces of salmon
    and sheets of pastry dough.

3 Brush the tops of the packages
    with melted butter and bake
    20 minutes. Serve with the
    remaining Sweet Chili Jelly.

sweet chili jelly

• • • • • • • • • • • • • • • • • • • •

makes about 1 pint

3 cooking apples, chopped (include the
    cores, peel, and pits)

1 handful fresh or frozen cranberries

2 fresh red chilies, finely chopped
½ red bell pepper, seeded and chopped
¾ cup plus 2 tablespoons red wine
    vinegar
¾ cup plus 2 tablespoons sugar

1 Put all the ingredients, except
    the sugar, and 7 ounces water
    in a pan, and bring to a boil.
    Lower the heat and simmer

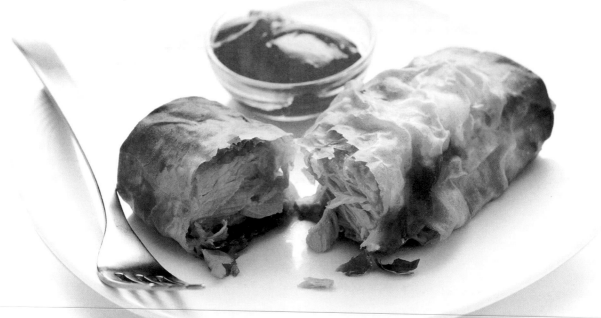

20 minutes, stirring occasionally. Leave to cool slightly. Mash the apple, adding more water, if necessary, for a slightly runny sauce.

2 Strain the sauce or drain it through a piece of cheesecloth suspended over a large bowl (this can take several hours). Pour more water through the pulp, if necessary, so you have 1 cup plus 2 tablespoons juice.

3 To make the jam, heat the juice with the sugar, stirring continuously until the sugar dissolves. Bring to a boil, then lower the heat and simmer slowly, skimming the surface, 10 minutes. Put a teaspoon of the jam on a cold plate and, when cool, press with a finger: if the surface wrinkles, the jelly is set. Remove from the heat, skim and leave to cool. Pour into a clean, dry 1-pint preserving jar. Seal and process in a water bath.

mild shrimp and coconut curry

serves 4

2 tablespoons olive oil
2 teaspoons mustard seeds
1 onion, finely chopped
1-inch piece gingerroot, peeled and finely chopped
2 garlic cloves, crushed
½ teaspoon turmeric
1 teaspoon ground coriander
2 bay leaves
1 or 2 green chilies, finely sliced (seed for gentler heat)
20 raw jumbo shrimp, shelled
1¾ cups coconut cream
Grated zest and juice of 2 limes
1 handful chopped cilantro

1 Heat the oil in a pan and sauté the mustard seeds 30 seconds. Add the onion and cook until soft. Add the ginger, garlic, turmeric, and coriander and stir-fry 1 minute.

2 Add the bay leaves, chilies, and 1¼ cups water and bring to a boil. Simmer slowly 1 minute before adding the shrimp. Simmer 4 minutes longer, or until the shrimp are cooked, then add the coconut cream, lime zest and juice, and cilantro. Warm through and serve.

mildly tikka fish

serves 4

1-inch piece gingeroot, peeled and finely chopped
4 garlic cloves, crushed
7 tablespoons yogurt with live cultures
2 tablespoons olive oil
2 teaspoon turmeric
1 fresh red chili, seeded and finely chopped
2 teaspoons cumin seeds
4 fish steaks, such as tuna

1 Make the tikka mixture by mixing all the ingredients, except the fish steaks, together. Coat the fish in the tikka mixture and then leave to marinate in the refrigerator at least 2 hours.

2 Broil or barbecue the fish 4 minutes per side, or until just cooked through.

left: thai salmon filo parcels served with sweet chilli jelly

mildly spiced broiled chicken

serves 4

4 chicken breast halves

For the marinade:
1 fresh red chili, seeded and chopped
1 onion, chopped
1 lemongrass stalk, trimmed and
    chopped
4 tablespoons olive oil
2 teaspoons dark brown sugar
Grated zest and juice of 1 unwaxed
    lemon
½ tespoon turmeric

1   Score the chicken breasts.
2   Put the marinade ingredients in
    a blender to make a paste. Coat
    the chicken with the paste and
    marinate at least 2 hours.
3   Barbecue or broil the chicken
    over high heat until it is cooked.

herby lamb and eggplant kabobs

serves 4

1 pound lean lamb neck tenderloin,
    cubed
1 eggplant, cubes

For the marinade:
4 tablespoon extra virgin olive oil
Grated zest and juice of 1 unwaxed
    lemon
2 garlic cloves, crushed
1 sprig rosemary, chopped
4 sprigs thyme, chopped
Freshly ground black pepper

1   Mix together the marinade
    ingredients, season with black
    pepper, and pour over the lamb
    and eggplant. Set aside and
    leave to marinate at least
    1 hour.
2   Thread the lamb and eggplants
    alternately onto 8 metal
    skewers, then barbecue or broil
    over high heat to seal the meat.
    Reduce the heat and continue
    cooking 10 minutes, basting
    and turning frequently.

cod in soy sauce

serves 4

4 tablespoons extra virgin olive oil
1 red onion, finely chopped
2 garlic cloves, crushed
1 fresh red chili, seeded and chopped
    (optional)
1-inch piece gingerroot, peeled and
    finely chopped
4 cod fillets
2 tomatoes, skinned and chopped
Grated zest and juice of 1 small
    unwaxed lemon
2 tablespoons dark soy sauce
1 tablespoon dark brown sugar
½ cucumber, thinly sliced
1 handful chopped parsley

1   Heat the olive oil in a pan and
    sauté the onion and garlic until
    soft. Add the chili and ginger.
2   Add the fish, followed by the
    tomatoes, lemon zest and juice,

soy sauce, and sugar. Simmer
until the fish is cooked through.
3   Put the fish on the cucumber,
    pour the sauce over the top,
    and sprinkle with parsley.

braised halibut with sweet peppers

serves 4

3 red bell peppers, halved and seeded
3 yellow bell peppers, halved and
seeded
6 garlic cloves
3 sprigs thyme
3 sprigs rosemary
1 handful basil leaves, chopped
5 tablespoons olive oil
4 halibut fillets
½ cup vegetable stock
1 handful chopped parsley
Freshly ground black pepper

1   Heat the oven to 400°F.
2   Put the pepper halves face
    down on a baking sheet.
    Sprinkle the garlic, thyme, and
    rosemary over the tops and
    bake about 25 minutes until the
    pepper skins start to blister.
3   Put the peppers in a bowl
    (discard the garlic and herbs),
    cover with plastic wrap, and
    leave them to steam as they
    cool, which makes peeling
    easier). When cool, peel the
    peppers and cut into strips.

4 Sauté the peppers with the basil and half the olive oil 3 minutes. Season well with black pepper and keep warm.

5 Shallow-fry the halibut with the remaining olive oil, skin-side down, 5 minutes until colored. Turn the fish over, cover with the vegetable stock and simmer 5 minutes longer, or until cooked through.

6 Put the fish on top of the peppers and season well. Sprinkle the parsley over the top and serve.

vegetable gratinée with basil and walnuts

serves 4

4 tablespoons extra virgin olive oil
2 medium eggplants, cut into slices lengthwise
4 zucchini, sliced lengthwise
1 pound baby spinach leaves, chopped
2 handfuls walnuts, coarsely chopped
1 cup mozzarella or cheddar cheese
1/3 cup grated Parmesan

For the sauce:
6 tomatoes, chopped
1 red bell pepper, seeded and chopped
2 tablespoons extra virgin olive oil
1 onion, chopped
2 garlic cloves, crushed
1 tablespoon tomato paste
1 handful chopped basil
Scant ½ cup dry white wine
Freshly ground black pepper

1 Heat the oven to 375°F.

2 Lightly brush a heavy pan with olive oil and fry the eggplant and zucchini slices until they start to color; drain well on paper towels.

3 Steam the spinach leaves until just wilted; drain well.

4 To make the sauce, puree the tomatoes and red pepper in a blender. Heat the olive oil in a pan and sauté the onion and garlic. Add the puree, tomato paste, basil, and white wine. Bring to a boil and simmer, stirring, until starting to thicken. Season well with black pepper.

5 Place alternating layers of eggplant and zucchini slices, sauce, and spinach in a baking dish. Top with the walnuts and grated cheese and bake 30 minutes.

mushroom and walnut roast

serves 4

2 tablespoons extra virgin olive oil
1 onion, finely chopped
2 garlic cloves, crushed
8 cremini mushrooms, chopped
2 cups finely chopped walnuts
2 cups fresh wholewheat bread crumbs
1 omega-3-enriched egg, beaten
3 parsnips, peeled, boiled, and mashed
4 tablespoons lowfat plain yogurt
1 handful chopped mixed herbs, such as basil, thyme, rosemary, and parsley
2/3 cup vegetable stock
Freshly ground black pepper

1 Heat the oven to 350°F.

2 Lightly brush a 9- x 5-inch bread pan with oil. Put the remaining oil in a pan and sauté the onion, garlic, and mushrooms. Mix together the walnuts, bread crumbs, and the egg.

3 Mash the parsnips with the yogurt and herbs. Add the egg, mushroom mixture, and stock, and season with black pepper.

4 Put in the bread pan, cover with foil, and bake 50 minutes. Leave to stand 10 minutes before turning out and slicing.

dessert recipes

chocolate cinnamon-pecan brownies

serves 4

3½ ounces bittersweet chocolate (70 percent cocoa solids)
1 stick unsalted butter, softened at room temperature
1¼ cups plus 2 tablespoons sugar
1 teaspoon vanilla extract
2 eggs, beaten
⅔ cup all-purpose flour
4 tablespoons unsweetened cocoa powder
1 teaspoon ground cinnamon
1 cup chopped pecans

1 Heat the oven to 350°F.
2 Gently melt the chocolate in a heatproof bowl over a pan of simmering water.
3 Beat the butter until soft and creamy. Add the sugar and vanilla extract and beat until fluffy. Gradually beat in the eggs, then sift the all-purpose flour, cocoa powder, and cinnamon over. Add the pecan nuts and melted chocolate and stir gently until thoroughly mixed.
4 Pour into a nonstick 8-inch square cake pan. Bake 30 minutes, or until a toothpick comes out clean. Cut into squares and serve warm.

figs in red wine

serves 4

1 cup plus 1 tablespoon soft light brown sugar
1 cup red wine
8 firm but ripe figs, peeled

1 Combine the sugar, wine, and 1¾ cups water in a pan and slowly bring to a simmer, stirring until the sugar dissolves. Add the figs, cover, and poach 8 minutes, or until tender.
2 Remove the figs with a perforated spoon and leave to cool. Continue to simmer the syrup 15 minutes longer to reduce the volume. Leave to cool slightly, then pour over the figs. Serve warm.

chocolate cinnamon-pecan brownies

plum, apple, and almond crumble

serves 4

14 ounces dark red or black plums,
  stoned and chopped
2 Red Delicious apples, cored and
  chopped
1 teaspoon ground cinnamon
1 teaspoon soft brown sugar (optional)

For the crumble topping:
$^2/_3$ cup wholewheat flour
2 tablespoons butter
1 teaspoon ground cinnamon
¼ cup Demerara sugar
$^1/_3$ cup almonds, chopped

1 Heat the oven to 400°F.
2 Mix all the filling ingredients
   together and put in a
   baking dish.
3 Rub the flour and butter
   together in a bowl with
   your fingers, then stir in the
   cinnamon, sugar, and almonds.
4 Sprinkle the crumble topping
   over the fruit and pat down
   firmly. Bake 40 minutes. Leave
   to rest 15 minutes before
   serving warm.

strawberries in balsamic vinegar with vanilla mascarpone

serves 4

1 pound 5 ounces strawberries, washed,
  hulled, and halved
$^2/_3$ cup aged balsamic vinegar
5 tablespoon dark brown sugar
1 vanilla bean
1¾ cups mascarpone cheese
1 handful mint leaves, chopped

1 Put the strawberries, balsamic
   vinegar and dark brown sugar
   in a bowl, and mix. Leave the
   fruit to marinate for 1 hour,
   stirring regularly.
2 Score the middle of the vanilla
   bean and scrape out the seeds.
   (Tip: put the scraped vanilla
   bean in a jar and cover with
   sugar to make vanilla-flavored
   sugar—you can use this to
   sprinkle over ripe strawberries
   in the future.) Mix the seeds
   with the mascarpone cheese
   and leave to infuse.
3 Serve the strawberries and
   mascarpone with the mint
   sprinkled on top.

mulled cranberry apples

serves 4

1 cup freshly squeezed orange juice
6 tablespoons strong ginger ale
1-inch piece gingerroot, peeled and
  chopped
1 cinnamon stick
1 star anise
4 red apples, cored and chopped
2 handfuls fresh or frozen cranberries
2 tablespoons golden sugar
Low fat ice cream, to serve

1 Put all the ingredients in a pan
   and bring to a boil, stirring until
   the sugar dissolves. Simmer
   gently 5 minutes, then remove
   from the heat and leave to cool.
2 Remove the star anise and
   cinnamon stick and serve with
   the ice cream.

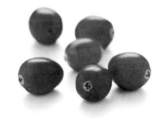

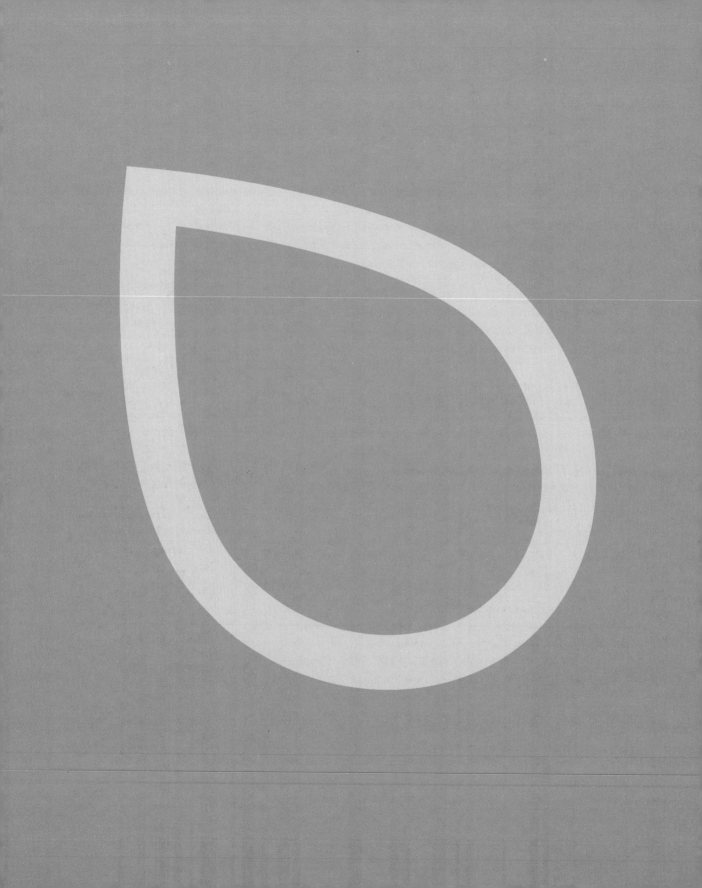

introducing the moderate program

The moderate program is a more advanced dietary and lifestyle plan for arthritis than the gentle program. It's designed for people whose joint pain, stiffness, and swelling remains troublesome, despite eating plenty of oily fish, nuts, fruit, and vegetables. The moderate program will help you recognize whether or not your symptoms are worsened by eating foods from the nightshade family of plants (see chart opposite).

The moderate program diet

The diet eliminates the foods from the nightshade family, as well as foods made with these foods, such as tomato ketchup, tomato paste, and Tabasco sauce. As described on page 51, these foods contain substances known as glycoalkaloids, which can worsen muscle and joint pain in some people (the reason for this is not fully understood). Some research suggests that eliminating nightshade plants from the diet can improve symptoms in 10 percent of people with arthritis of various types—others suggest it can help as many as 70 percent of people with arthritis.

Eat fruit, vegetables, nuts, and fish The diet contains plenty of non-nightshade fruit and vegetables that are rich in antioxidants, vitamins, and minerals. In particular, I encourage you to drink unsweetened apple juice and to eat fish, apples, Brazil nuts (for their rich selenium content), and macadamia nuts. With a delicious mild, crunchy flavor, macadamias contain as much as 75 percent oil, which has the highest content of monounsaturated fat found in nature.

Members of the nightshade (Solanaceae) family

food	botanical name
Eggplant	Solanum melongena
Bell peppers	Capsicum annuum
Cape gooseberry (ground cherry)	Physalis peruviana, P. ixocarpa
Garden huckleberry	Solanum melanocerasum
Habanero peppers	Capsicum chinense
Naranjillas	Solanum quitoense
Paprika/cayenne	Capsicum annuum (dried)
Pepinos	Solanum muricatum
Potato	Solanum tuberosum
Tabasco peppers	Capsicum frutescens
Tamarillo	Solanum betaceum
Tomatillo	Physalis philadelphica
Tomato	Solanum esculentum / Lycopersicon esculentum
Tobacco	Nicotiana tabacum (see the box on page 65 for advice on quitting smoking)

Shopping list

The following list shows you the non-nightshade foods you can eat on the moderate program. Base your shopping lists on these items, which feature in the recipes and eating plans.

drinks
apple juice (unsweetened), mineral water (low sodium), wine (red and dry white) teas: fruit; green, black, or white; herbal

dairy products
butter (unsalted), crème fraîche, fromage blanc (lowfat), heavy cream, milk (lowfat and nonfat), yogurt (plain lowfat with live cultures and Greek yogurt) cheeses: blue, cheddar, cottage cheese (plain, with chives, pineapple), dolcelatte, Gorgonzola, haloumi, mozzarella, Parmesan, pecorino, Roquefort (select lowfat versions)

fruit
apples (especially Red Delicious and cooking), apricots (fresh and semidried), bananas, blackberries, blueberries, dates, figs (fresh and dried), grapefruit (blond, pink, red; see caution on page 83), grapes (green, red, purple), guava, kiwifruit, lemons, mango, oranges, papaya, peaches, pears, pineapple, plums, pomegranate, prunes, raisins, raspberries, strawberries, watermelon

vegetables
arugula, avocados, bean sprouts, beets, black beans, broccoli, butternut squash, cabbage (red and green), carrots, celery, celery root, chickpeas, corn, cucumber, Florence fennel, green beans, lentils (red, green), mixed salad leaves, mushrooms, onions (baby, white, red), pumpkin, radish, scallions, spinach, sprouted beans, sweet potatoes, watercress, zucchini

nuts and seeds
almonds, hazelnuts, macadamias, pecans, pistachios, pumpkin seeds, sesame seeds, walnuts

herbs, spices, oils, and vinegar
basil, bay leaves, black pepper (freshly ground), chives, cilantro, cinnamon (sticks and ground), cloves (whole and ground), coriander, cumin, dill, fennel, garlic, mint, nutmeg, oregano/marjoram, parsley, peppercorns (black, green, red), rosemary, sage, tarragon, thyme, turmeric; extra virgin olive oil (for drizzling and dressings), olive oil (for cooking), macadamia nut oil, walnut oil; red wine vinegar, white wine vinegar

grains
coarse Scotch oats, fresh and dried pasta (wholewheat and hemp), high-fiber breakfast cereals, muesli (unsweetened), oatmeal, rice (brown, red, risotto), rice noodles, quinoa, specialty breads (ciabatta and focaccia), rye bread, wheat flour (all-purpose) or similar, wholewheat/multigrain bread and rolls, wholewheat pita bread, wild rice

proteins
omega-3-enriched eggs; fish: anchovy, bream, haddock (smoked, no colorings), herring, mackerel, mullet (gray), salmon (fresh and smoked), shrimp, red snapper, sea bass, trout (fresh and smoked), tuna (fresh and canned in olive oil); meat: lean bacon, chicken, pork chops

miscellaneous
bouillon cubes (beef, chicken, or vegetable), black olives, bittersweet chocolate (70 percent cocoa solids), hummus, mayonnaise, mustard (wholegrain), olive oil spread, runny honey, sugar (granulated and dark and soft brown), vanilla extract

Dessert recipes Some of the dessert recipes are more decadent than usually found in my Natural Health Guru books. For example, Cinnamon-Chocolate Nut Terrine (see page 140) includes heavy cream and sugar, and the Raspberry and Red Wine Sorbet (see page 139) includes red wine and sugar. This is justified during the moderate program in that, nutritionally, the other ingredients are extremely healthy. (Also, red wine and bittersweet chocolate are rich in antioxidants.) My primary aim is simply to test whether or not your problems are linked to the consumption of nightshade glycoalkaloids. If you prefer to omit cream, sugar, and alcohol from your diet, replace richer dishes with fruit or eat approximately 1½ ounces bittersweet chocolate (at least 70 percent cocoa solids) by itself.

Drinking plenty of fluids As with all the programs, you need to drink plenty of fluids to hydrate your joints. Keep a small bottle of water or cold herbal tea, such as ginger tea, with you at all times, and sip it regularly throughout the day, especially in hot weather or if you are more active. Remember that by the time you feel thirsty, you are already dehydrated.

Losing weight Although the moderate program is not designed for weight loss, you should lose any excess weight slowly and naturally as a result of eating healthily. If you need to lose weight, you can enhance the process by eating smaller portions, especially of starchy foods, such as pasta, bread, and rice. Also, omit the dessert recipes that include sugar and cream.

The moderate program exercise routine

The exercise program gives you a series of stretches that will improve your joint flexibility. Repeat these once or twice a day, adding each day's exercise onto the previous one/s. In addition, you should aim to do brisk aerobic exercise, ideally for at least 20 minutes

The moderate program supplements

These are the supplements I think are most important to take on the moderate program—higher doses are suggested than for the gentle program. Read about these supplements on pages 58–63 to help you decide which you want to take. You can, of course, take all of them, as I have designed this plan to include supplements with the best synergistic action. Supplements are widely available in drug stores, supermarkets, and healthfood stores.

recommended daily supplements

- Chondroitin (1,200 mg)
- Glucosamine sulfate (1,500 mg)
- Vitamin C (1000 mg)
- Omega-3 fish oils (600 mg daily, for example 2 x 1 g fish oil capsules, each supplying 180 mg EPA + 120 mg DHA)
- Evening primrose oil (1000 mg)

optional daily supplements (these provide additional benefits)

- Vitamin-B complex (50 mg)
- Vitamin D (10 mcg)
- Vitamin E (400 iu/268 mg)
- Calcium (500 mg)
- Selenium (100 mcg)
- Green-lipped mussel extracts (400–600 mg)
- Garlic—especially if you have rheumatoid arthritis (supplying 1000 mcg allicin)
- MSM (1 g)

per day. Use heat and ice, as explained on page 31 to help prepare your joints for exercise, and to treat them afterward, if necessary. Walking and cycling are both good options for the moderate program. Cycling is especially good for your hips, knees, and ankles, as it flexes and extends these joints without the burden of carrying your weight. Here's a suggested regime to help you slowly increase the amount of exercise you do over the following two months. Remember to warm up and cool down.

- Weeks one and two: walk or cycle 15 minutes on Tuesday, Thursday, and Saturday.
- Week three: walk or cycle 15 minutes on Thursday and 20 minutes on Tuesday and Saturday.
- Weeks four and five: walk or cycle 20 minutes on Tuesday, Thursday, Saturday, and Sunday.
- Week six: walk or cycle 20 minutes on Tuesday and Saturday and 25 minutes on Thursday and Sunday.
- Week seven: walk or cycle 25 minutes on Tuesday, Thursday, Saturday, and Sunday.
- Week eight: walk or cycle 25 minutes on Tuesday and Saturday and 30 minutes on Thursday and Sunday.

The moderate program therapies

During this program I show you some hand reflexology techniques you can do at home followed by some techniques from other therapies. Please now book an appointment for a reflexology massage (see day seven) and to see a chiropractor (see day fourteen).

1

the moderate program day one

Daily menu

- **Breakfast: Green Tea Compote (see page 132). One slice of toast**

- **Morning snack: an apple**

- **Lunch: Pear, Avocado, and Blue Cheese Salad (see page 134). Wholewheat bread roll. Lowfat yogurt with live cultures with a handful of black or red grapes or berries**

- **Afternoon snack: handful of macadamias**

- **Dinner: Pasta with Smoked Salmon and Fennel (see page 139). Green salad drizzled with Macadamia Nut and Lemon Juice Dressing (see page 137). Fresh fruit, such as plums**

- **Drinks: 2½ cups lowfat or nonfat milk. Unlimited tea (including herbal or fruit tea) and mineral water. Glass of apple juice**

- **Supplements: see page 113**

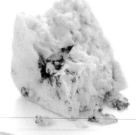

The exercises I describe over the following two weeks incorporate stretches with "range-of-motion" movements to help strengthen your muscles and maintain joint flexibility. Repeat these once or twice a day, adding each day's exercise to the previous one(s) so you build up a stretch sequence.

Daily exercise routine

Start a walking or cycling regime, as explained on pages 112–113. Also do this simple jaw exercise.

Jaw exercise

1 Say your vowels by opening your mouth as wide as you can and stretching your jaw muscles in an exaggerated way: "A ... E ... I ... O ... U."
2 Do this five times.

Reflexology

Hand reflexology is beneficial for joints throughout your body.

Hand massage 1

1 Using an aromatherapy hand cream, such as one that contains ginger essential oil, lightly massage between the tendons on the back of your left

hand, working from your wrist to your fingers.
2 Gently massage the webbing between your fingers, and between your finger and thumb, to improve lymph circulation throughout the body, remove toxins, and reduce inflammation.
3 After one or two minutes, gently squeeze the bottom of your thumb and slide your massaging fingers and thumb toward its tip. When you reach the bottom of the nail, gently squeeze the nail and slide your hand off the tip. Do this with each finger. Now repeat the massage on your other hand.

Know your sensitivities

You might find certain foods in the moderate program seem to worsen your symptoms —even recognized arthritis superfoods. Avoid any foods to which you know you're sensitive (for example, acid-forming foods, see pages 52–53) and replace them with alternatives.

day two

Daily menu

- **Breakfast: Apple, Kiwifruit, and Watercress Smoothie (see page 132)**

- **Morning snack: an apple**

- **Lunch: hummus with sticks of raw carrot, celery, radish, and scallion. Foccacia bread. Lowfat yogurt with live cultures with a handful of black or red grapes or berries**

- **Afternoon snack: handful of Brazil nuts**

- **Dinner: Herby Pecan Nut Roast (see page 135). Quinoa. Spinach. Carrots. Cinnamon-Chocolate Nut Terrine (see page 140).**

- **Drinks: 2½ cups lowfat or nonfat milk. Unlimited tea (including herbal or fruit tea) and mineral water. Glass of apple juice**

- **Supplements: see page 113**

Daily exercise routine

Continue with your walking or cycling regime, as described on pages 112–113. Add the following stretch to yesterday's jaw exercise.

Neck circles

1 Tilt your head to the right as if trying to rest your ear on your shoulder. Keep your shoulders relaxed and down.

2 Slowly circle your head forward so your chin is near to your chest. Keep circling it around so your left ear is as near as possible to your left shoulder. Finally, tilt your head back to complete the circle. Do five more circles.

Reflexology

Today, you're going to stimulate the solar plexus area at the top of your palm—it's situated a thumb's width below your middle finger on each side.

Hand massage 2

1 Apply pressure to the solar plexus point with your thumb and gradually push harder until you reach the limit of comfort.

Hold the pressure on this reflex at least 20 seconds, then press and release in quick pulses of one or two seconds.

2 Now gently massage across the upper palm beneath your remaining fingers, to stimulate the diaphragm line.

3 Then, as yesterday, gently squeeze the base of the thumb and slide your massaging fingers and thumb toward the tip. When you reach the base of the nail, gently squeeze the nail and slide your hand off the tip. Repeat with each finger. Now do the same with your other hand.

Know your pain limits

If today's neck circles hurt or make you feel dizzy, stop. The same applies to any other exercise. You should always exercise without pain, or within the limits of mild pain. If you're concerned, ask your doctor for advice on what type of exercise suits you best.

the moderate program
day three

Daily menu

- **Breakfast: Fresh Figs with Blueberries (see page 132)**

- **Morning snack: an apple**

- **Lunch: grated beets (cooked or raw), carrot, cheddar cheese, and zucchini arranged in four piles on a bed of mixed lettuce leaves. Wholewheat pita bread. Lowfat yogurt with live cultures with a handful of black or red grapes or berries**

- **Afternoon snack: handful of macadamias**

- **Dinner: Baked Whole Fish with Lemon and Herbs (see page 137). Wild rice. Green salad leaves drizzled with Macadamia Nut and Lemon Juice Dressing (see page 137). Baked banana**

- **Drinks: 2½ cups lowfat or nonfat milk. Unlimited tea (including herbal or fruit tea) and mineral water. Glass of apple juice**

- **Supplements: see page 113**

To make today's dinner dessert, wrap a peeled banana in foil and bake in a medium oven, alongside the fish, 20 minutes. Serve with crème fraîche.

Daily exercise routine

Continue with your walking or cycling regime, as described on pages 112–113. Add the following stretch to your daily sequence.

Shoulder shrugs

1 Stand comfortably, feet apart and your arms by your sides.
2 Lift your shoulders as high as you can and keep them there for a count of three. Then relax.
3 Repeat five to 10 times.

Reflexology

Repeat yesterday's hand massage, then I'd like you to concentrate on your spinal reflexes. These run along the outer side of your thumb, with the cervical area starting level with the base of your nail, followed by the thoracic spine, then the lumbar region in the curve where your hand and wrist meet, then the sacrum and coccyx at the side of your wrist (see diagram, page 38).

Hand massage 3

1 Gently press along the outer side of your thumb to see if you can find areas that feel gritty or tender. Focus on these by gradually pressing harder until you reach the limit of comfort.
2 Hold the pressure for at least 20 seconds, then press and release in quick pulses of one or two seconds.
3 As before, gently squeeze the base of your thumb and then slide your massaging thumb and fingers toward the top. At the bottom of the nail, gently squeeze and slide your fingers off the tip. Repeat with each finger. Now do the same with your other hand.

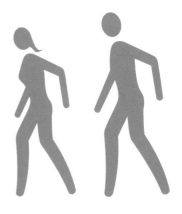

day four

Daily menu

- **Breakfast: Omega-3 Omelet with Smoked Trout and Tarragon (see page 132)**

- **Morning snack: an apple**

- **Lunch: Lentil, Sweet Potato, and Apricot Soup (see page 135). Wholewheat bread roll. Lowfat yogurt with live cultures with a handful of black or red grapes or berries**

- **Afternoon snack: handful of Brazil nuts**

- **Dinner: roast chicken. Braised Red Cabbage with Apple and Red Wine (see page 135). Celery Root Puree (see right). Broccoli. Fresh fruit, such as mango**

- **Drinks: 2½ cups lowfat or nonfat milk. Unlimited herbal or green, black, or white tea and mineral water. Glass of apple juice**

- **Supplements: see page 113**

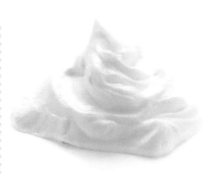

Celery root puree is a delicious side dish that's an excellent alternative to potatoes. To make it, boil celery root 25 minutes, or until it's soft. Puree it in a food processor and then stir in crème fraîche or lowfat plain yogurt with live cultures and lots of black pepper. Add nutmeg and parsley.

Daily exercise routine

Keep up your walking or cycling regime (see pages 112–113). Do the stretch exercises from days one to three, then add in the following shoulder rolls.

Shoulder rolls

1 Stand comfortably with your feet apart. Let both arms hang down by your sides. Slowly circle one shoulder forward and upward, then backward and downward.

2 Do this five to 10 times on both shoulders, making the rolls progressively faster.

Reflexology

Repeat yesterday's hand massage, then, after stimulating the spinal reflexes, I'd like you to move onto the sacroiliac joint reflex. This is situated on the back of each hand, just above the wrist crease and in line with your ring finger (see the diagram on page 38).

Hand massage 4

1 Gently massage the sacroiliac joint reflex. If it feels tender, increase the pressure until you reach the limit of comfort. Hold this pressure for at least 20 seconds, then press and release in quick pulses of one or two seconds.

2 As before, finish the massage by gently squeezing the bottom of your thumb and sliding your massaging thumb and fingers toward its top. When you reach the bottom of the nail, gently squeeze and slide your fingers off the tip. Repeat with each finger. Now do the same with your other hand.

the moderate program day five

Daily menu

- **Breakfast: muesli (or similar high-fiber cereal with dried fruit) and lowfat or nonfat milk**

- **Morning snack: an apple**

- **Lunch: avocado and shrimp open sandwich on rye bread with a scraping of olive-oil spread. Lowfat yogurt with live cultures with a handful of black or red grapes or berries**

- **Afternoon snack: handful of macadamias**

- **Dinner: Oaty Mackerel with Beet Salsa (see page 136). Mashed sweet potato. Green salad leaves drizzled with Macadamia Nut and Lemon Juice Dressing (see page 137). Raspberry and Red Wine Sorbet (see page 139)**

- **Drinks: 2½ cups lowfat or nonfat milk. Unlimited tea (including herbal or fruit tea) and mineral water. Glass of apple juice**

- **Supplements: see page 113**

Although you can't eat some of the hotter spices, such as chili, on the moderate program, you can continue to eat black pepper (*Piper nigrum*). This doesn't belong to the nightshade family, so therefore doesn't contain glycoalkaloids that can upset your arthritis.

Daily exercise routine

Continue with your walking or cycling regime, as described on pages 112–113. Do the stretches from days one to four, then add the following.

Arm bends

1 Tuck your hands (or just your thumbs) into your armpits. Rotate your arms so your elbows move in large circles.
2 Repeat five to 10 times.

Reflexology

Repeat yesterday's hand reflexology massage. After stimulating the sacroiliac joint reflexes, please move onto the hip reflexes. These are situated on the edge of each hand at the base of the little finger (see the diagram on page 38).

Sweet potatoes

Today's dinner includes mashed sweet potato (please don't substitute normal potatoes, because these are members of the Solanaceae family). Sweet potato is not only more flavorsome than its regular counterpart, it's also a rich source of antioxidant carotenoids, many of which are converted into vitamin A in the body.

Hand massage 5

1 Gently massage the hip reflex on your hand. If it's tender, increase the pressure up to the limit of comfort. Hold at least 20 seconds, then press and release in quick pulses of one or two seconds.
2 Gently squeeze the bottom of the thumb and slide your massaging thumb and fingers toward the top. When you reach the bottom of the nail, gently squeeze and then slide your hand off the tip. Repeat with each finger. Now do the same with your other hand.

day six

Daily menu

- **Breakfast: half a grapefruit. Toast and broiled bacon**

- **Morning snack: an apple**

- **Lunch: bowl of mixed salad leaves drizzled with Macadamia Nut and Lemon Juice Dressing (see page 137). Cottage cheese with pineapple and grated beets. Ciabatta bread**

- **Afternoon snack: handful of Brazil nuts**

- **Dinner: Pasta with Pesto Sauce (see page 138). Green salad drizzled with Macadamia Nut and Lemon Juice Dressing (see page 137) and sprinkled with shavings of Parmesan cheese and mixed seeds. Berry and Hazelnut Meringue (see page 140)**

- **Drinks: 2½ cups lowfat or nonfat milk. Unlimited tea (including herbal or fruit tea) and mineral water. Glass of apple juice**

- **Supplements: see page 113**

Tomorrow's lunch is cold pasta and pesto salad. Prepare in advance by cooking extra pasta for today's dinner and storing it in the fridge.

Daily exercise routine

Continue walking or cycling as outlined on pages 112–113. Do the stretch exercises from days one to five, then add the following.

Arm circles

1 Raise your right arm out to your side and slowly swing it around to draw a circle in the air.

2 Do this five to 10 times, then repeat with your left arm.

Reflexology

Repeat yesterday's hand reflexology massage, then after stimulating the hip reflexes, I'd like you to move onto the knee reflexes. These are on the edge of each hand at the bottom of the little finger just above the hip reflexes (see page 38).

Hand massage 6

1 Gently massage your knee reflex. If the point feels tender, increase the pressure until

you reach the limit of comfort. Maintain the pressure for at least 20 seconds, then press and release in quick pulses of one or two seconds.

2 Finish the massage in the usual way: gently squeeze the bottom of the thumb and slide your massaging thumb and fingers toward the top. When you reach the bottom of the nail, gently squeeze and slide your fingers off the tip. Repeat with each finger. Do the same with your other hand.

Red meat and arthritis

Some people find eating red meat worsens their arthritis. If your joint pains flare up over the next few days, this might be related to the bacon in today's menu. If you suspect meat activates your symptoms, avoid meat for the rest of this program, substituting vegetarian dishes instead. (Don't include tomatoes, potatoes, eggplants, or bell peppers in your meals).

the moderate program day seven

Daily menu

- **Breakfast: fruit platter: one chopped orange, one slice of watermelon, one sliced kiwifruit, and some chopped mango. A selection of lowfat cheeses. A slice of wholewheat bread**

- **Morning snack: an apple**

- **Lunch: pasta with pesto (from yesterday). Bowl of mixed green salad leaves with sprouted beans, fennel, and celery, drizzled with Macadamia Nut and Lemon Juice Dressing (see page 137). Lowfat yogurt with live cultures with a handful of black or red grapes**

- **Afternoon snack: handful of macadamias**

- **Dinner: Marinated Herring (see page 136). Green salad drizzled with Macadamia Nut and Lemon Juice Dressing (see page 137). Corn. Brown rice. Fresh fruit, such as papaya**

- **Drinks: 2½ cups lowfat or nonfat milk. Unlimited tea (including herbal or fruit tea) and mineral water. Glass of apple juice**

- **Supplements: see page 113**

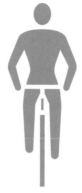

Daily exercise routine

Keep up your walking or cycling routine (see pages 112–113). Do the six exercises in your stretch sequence so far and then add today's stretch.

Arm windmills

1 Stand comfortably with your feet apart and your arms by your sides. Lift both arms forward and up, keeping them straight until they are high above your head. Then spread your arms out sideways and move them down to complete a full circle.

2 Repeat this windmill movement five to 10 times. Now do the same movements in the opposite direction five to 10 times.

Consulting a reflexologist

After following the moderate program for one week, you should have started to notice an improvement in your arthritis symptoms. I suggest you now visit a reflexologist. Book yourself in for four weekly sessions. Over the past week, you have learned some basic reflexology techniques that are beneficial for people with arthritis—a reflexologist will be able to show you additional techniques to use. Most reflexologists work on reflexes in the feet, but some may use reflexes on your hands or ears, too. After removing your footwear, you will be asked to relax on a seat or couch with your feet raised. The therapist will lightly dust your feet with powder and will then massage your reflexes using their fingers and thumbs. Reflexologists focus on areas of tenderness and grittiness to diagnose distant problems in the body and will stimulate specific points to open up blocked nerve pathways and promote the flow of energy. A session usually lasts from 45 to 60 minutes. To find a reflexologist, check the resources on pages 175.

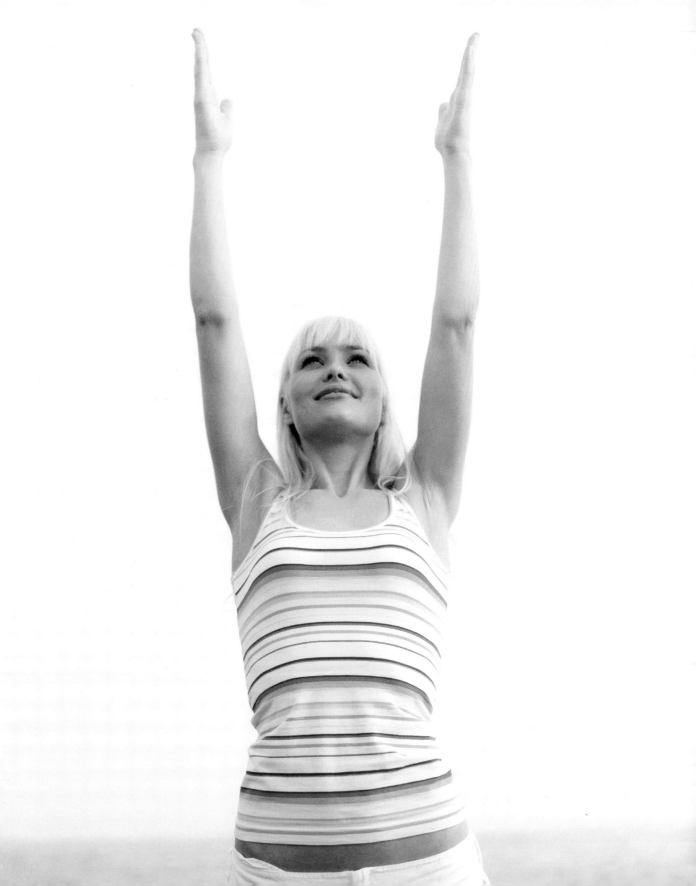

the moderate program day eight

Daily menu

- **Breakfast: Green Tea Compote (see page 132). One slice of wholewheat toast**

- **Morning snack: an apple**

- **Lunch: Tuna, Pomegranate, and Anchovy Salad (see page 133). Wholewheat pita bread. Lowfat yogurt with live cultures with a handful of black or red grapes or berries**

- **Afternoon snack: handful of Brazil nuts**

- **Dinner: Pasta with Walnuts and Cilantro (see page 138). Bowl of green salad leaves drizzled with Macadamia Nut and Lemon Juice Dressing (see page 137). Fresh fruit, such as an orange**

- **Drinks: 2½ cups lowfat or nonfat milk. Unlimited tea (including herbal or fruit tea) and mineral water. Glass of apple juice**

- **Supplements: see page 113**

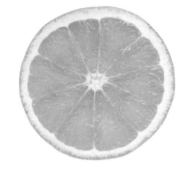

Over the next few days I introduce several complementary therapies that can be beneficial for arthritis. Once you've found a therapy that suits you, try to find other ways to incorporate it into your daily routine.

Daily exercise routine

Continue with your walking or cycling regime, as outlined on pages 112–113. Do the stretches you've learned so far, and then add these wrist rotations.

Wrist circling

1 Place your palms and forearms flat on a table. Rotate your wrists so your palms turn to face upward. Try to rotate them to the point at which the backs of your hands come to rest on the table.

2 Rotate your hands back to the starting position and repeat five to 10 times.

Herbalism

Today, I'd like you to start using herbalism to help your arthritis symptoms. The remedy I've selected as most appropriate for the moderate program is ginger, which helps to suppress the release of inflammatory substances within joints. Read about it on page 28 to confirm it is suitable for you. Start taking a ginger supplement supplying at least 300 mg once or twice a day, depending on the severity of your symptoms. Choose a brand offering about 15 mg gingerols (the active ingredient) per capsule.

Staying warm
Making sure you stay warm and avoid cold drafts are simple, but effective, ways to reduce joint pain. Taking frequent hot baths or showers can also be helpful to ease joint symptoms.

day nine

Daily menu

- **Breakfast: Apple, Kiwi, and Watercress Smoothie (see page 132)**

- **Morning snack: an apple**

- **Lunch: Pear, Avocado, and Blue Cheese Salad (see page 134). Focaccia bread. Lowfat yogurt with live cultures with a handful of black or red grapes or berries**

- **Afternoon snack: handful of macadamias**

- **Dinner: Baked Whole Fish with Lemon and Herbs (see page 137). Baked pumpkin, butternut squash, or sweet potato. Red rice. Baked Apples with Cloves (see page 139)**

- **Drinks: 2½ cups lowfat or nonfat milk. Unlimited tea (including herbal or fruit tea) and mineral water. Glass of apple juice**

- **Supplements: see page 113**

Ideally you should be doing 15 minutes of aerobic exercise three times a week. Any exercise is better than none, however, so if 15 minutes is difficult, do what you can. Even pottering around the house is good for your joints.

Daily exercise routine

Keep walking or cycling (see pages 112–113). Do the stretch exercises from days one to eight, then add the following finger-strengthening exercise.

Finger flexes

1 Squeeze a soft foam ball in the palm of one hand by clenching your fingers as tightly as possible. Hold for a count of five, then relax.
2 Do this for one minute, then repeat with the other hand.

Copper therapy

Today, I'd like you to buy a copper bracelet and wear it continuously for at least the remainder of this program. As described on page 33, copper has the potential to reduce joint pains in people who are copper deficient.

Stay hydrated

Drink at least 2 quarts fluid per day to maintain good hydration and a good flow of nutrients to your joints. Choose a brand of mineral water that's rich in calcium —an important mineral for bone health. As well as water, drink fruit or herbal teas. Soup counts toward your fluid intake, too.

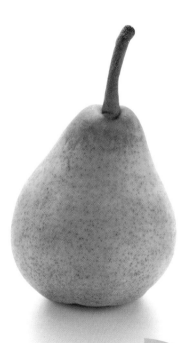

the moderate program
day ten

Daily menu

- **Breakfast: oatmeal made with rolled oats and sprinkled with chopped banana and slivered almonds**

- **Morning snack: an apple**

- **Lunch: Avocado and Smoked Salmon Oriental Salad (see page 133). Wholewheat bread roll. Lowfat yogurt with live cultures with a handful of black or red grapes or berries**

- **Afternoon snack: handful of Brazil nuts**

- **Dinner: Herby Pecan Nut Roast (see page 135). Roast baby onions. Roast mushrooms. Green beans. Hemp pasta drizzled with olive oil. Fresh fruit, such as guava**

- **Drinks: 2½ cups lowfat or nonfat milk. Unlimited tea (including herbal or fruit tea) and mineral water. Glass of apple juice**

- **Supplements: see page 113**

Daily exercise routine

Continue to walk or cycle (see pages 112–113). Do the nine stretch exercises you've learned so far and then add the following waist exercises.

Waist twists

1 Stand comfortably, feet slightly apart. Link your hands and stretch your arms straight out in front. Without moving your hips, swivel smoothly to the left by twisting your waist.
2 When you have twisted as far as you can, hold your position for a count of three, then return to face forward.
3 Repeat the twist to the right. Repeat the whole exercise five to 10 times.

Herbalism

Today, I'd like you to buy a herbal preparation of arnica gel to rub into your affected joints. Apply the gel two or three times a day for at least the next five days.

Laughing therapy

Laughing is an excellent preventative measure for joint and back pains. It acts as an antidote to stress and helps you relax. (Stress, on the other hand, causes clenching of muscles and tension, especially in the back area.) Laughter also enhances general well-being.

Note that herbal arnica gel contains between one and 25 percent *Arnica montana* extract. This contains helenalin and related compounds, which have an analgesic, anti-inflammatory action. In contrast, the homeopathic arnica gel that you may have used in the gentle program (see page 93) is prepared using the principles of homeopathy and contains no measurable amount of arnica. Make sure you choose the herbal preparation of arnica today.

the moderate program day eleven

Daily menu

- **Breakfast: Fresh Figs with Blueberries (see page 132)**

- **Morning snack: an apple**

- **Lunch: Lentil, Sweet Potato, and Apricot Soup (see page 134). Wholewheat bread roll. Lowfat yogurt with live cultures with a handful of black or red grapes or berries**

- **Afternoon snack: handful of macadamia nuts**

- **Dinner: Smoked Haddock Omelet with Béchamel Sauce (see page 136). Bowl of green salad leaves drizzled with Macadamia Nut and Lemon Juice Dressing (see page 137). Fresh fruit, such as a banana**

- **Drinks: 2½ cups lowfat or nonfat milk. Unlimited tea (including herbal or fruit tea) and mineral water. Glass of apple juice**

- **Supplements: see page 113**

Macadamia nuts and their oil feature almost every day in the moderate program. This is because they have strong antioxidant properties that helps to reduce inflammation in the body. Macadamia nut oil has a higher percentage of monounsaturated fat than other oils—81 percent compared to 73 percent for olive oil, 62 percent for avocado oil, and 60 percent for canola oil.

Daily exercise routine

Continue with your walking or cycling regime, as outlined on pages 112–113. Do the stretch exercises from days one to 10, then add these ankle exercises.

Ankle rotations

1 Stand comfortably with one hand on a table for support. Lift one foot and rotate the ankle in

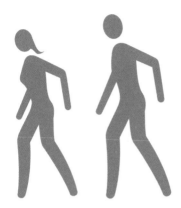

10 complete circles clockwise then anticlockwise.

2 Repeat with the other foot.

Magnetic therapy

Today, I'd like you to apply a magnetic wrap around your most painful joint. This helps to improve circulation, warms the joint, promotes healing, and reduces pain. Magnetic wraps are widely available from drug stores, healthfood stores, and online sites.

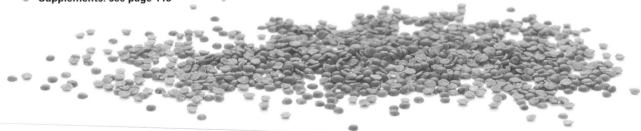

day twelve

Daily menu

- **Breakfast: muesli (or similar high-fiber cereal with fruit) with lowfat or nonfat milk**

- **Morning snack: an apple**

- **Lunch: Waldorf Salad (see opposite) on a bed of mixed green salad leaves. Ciabatta bread. Lowfat yogurt with live cultures with a handful of black or red grapes or berries**

- **Afternoon snack: handful of Brazil nuts**

- **Dinner: pork chop with rice and Delicious Black Beans (see page 138). Broccoli. Chocolate Lava Pudding (see page 140)**

- **Drinks: 2½ cups lowfat or nonfat milk. Unlimited tea (including herbal or fruit tea) and mineral water. Glass of apple juice**

- **Supplements: see page 113**

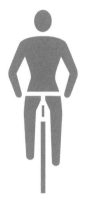

To make the Waldorf Salad for today's lunch simply mix chopped apple, celery, and walnuts with lowfat mayonnaise. If you're trying to lose weight, omit the ciabatta bread from your lunch and, at dinner time, eat fruit for dessert instead of the Chocolate Lava Pudding. Alternatively, if you want to get the antioxidant benefits of bittersweet chocolate without too many extra calories eat about 1½ ounces on its own.

Daily exercise routine

Continue to walk or cycle (see pages 112–113). Do the stretch exercises from days one to eleven, then add the following knee bends to your routine.

Mattress support

Check that your mattress is not too old and saggy—ideally, you should change it every five to 10 years, depending on its quality. Invest in a "memory foam" mattress, if you can afford it (see page 64).

Knee bends

1 Stand with your feet apart and your knees slightly bent. Put your hands on your knees. Bend your knees up and down. Don't make them completely straight and don't let your bottom go below your knees.

2 Do this five to 10 times.

Homeopathy

Try one of the remedies shown on page 32. Select the one that most accurately describes your condition. Take a 6 c potency remedy twice a day for five days. Alternatively, if you consulted a homeopath after finishing the gentle program, continue with the remedies he or she prescribed.

the moderate program day thirteen

Daily menu

- **Breakfast: half a grapefruit (see caution on page 83). One slice of wholewheat toast. Mushrooms and garlic sautéed in olive oil**

- **Morning snack: an apple**

- **Lunch: Spicy Sweet Potato Salad (see page 134). Lowfat yogurt with live cultures with a handful of black or red grapes or berries**

- **Afternoon snack: handful of macadamias**

- **Dinner: Pesto and Tuna Ciabatta Pizzas (see page 138). Green salad drizzled with Macadamia Nut and Lemon Juice Dressing (see page 137). Fresh fruit, such as a banana**

- **Drinks: 2½ cups lowfat or nonfat milk. Unlimited tea (including herbal or fruit tea) and mineral water. Glass of apple juice**

- **Supplements: see page 113**

You can avoid stress on your hand joints by holding objects loosely and using arthritis aids, such as faucet grips, to help you turn faucets on and off, and especially designed doorknobs that don't need to be turned or twisted. Try to hold objects in your palm rather than with your fingers, and use two hands instead of one.

Daily exercise routine

Go cycling or walking as described on pages 112–113. Do the stretch exercises you've learned so far and then add the following heel and toe lifts.

Heel and toe lifts

1 Start in the position you were in for yesterday's exercise (leaning forward with your hands on your knees). Lift both heels off the floor, so your calf muscles strongly contract.

Lower your heels then lift your toes up toward your shins.

2 Repeat five to 10 times.

Meditation

Today, I'd like you to try a crystal meditation that will help you relax and will reduce pain in a particular joint. Crystals are believed to amplify the power of meditation. Choose a piece of amethyst or clear rock quartz, or another crystal you feel particularly drawn to.

Crystal meditation

1 Sit comfortably in a chair with your eyes shut. Hold your crystal in both hands on your lap. Clear your mind of thoughts by focusing your attention on the crystal.

2 Visualize healing energy passing through the crystal and concentrating in your painful joint(s). Do this for 15 minutes.

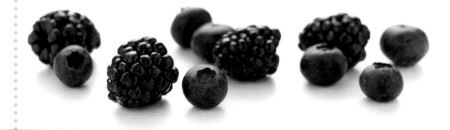

day fourteen

Daily menu

- **Breakfast: Herring with Oatmeal and Pecan Nuts (see page 132).**

- **Morning snack: an apple**

- **Lunch: buffalo mozzarella and sliced mango open sandwich on rye bread with a scraping of olive-oil spread. Lowfat yogurt with live cultures with a handful of black or red grapes or berries**

- **Afternoon snack: handful of Brazil nuts**

- **Dinner: risotto made with wild mushrooms (see box). Green salad drizzled with Macadamia Nut and Lemon Juice Dressing (see page 137). Fresh fruit, such as a peach**

- **Drinks: 2½ cups lowfat or nonfat milk. Unlimited tea (including herbal or fruit tea) and mineral water. Glass of apple juice**

- **Supplements: see page 113**

Daily exercise routine

Continue to walk or cycle (see pages 112–113). Do the stretch exercises from days one to thirteen, then finish with this shaking exercise.

Arm and leg shakes

1 Shake each hand and arm in turn for a minute or two.
2 Repeat with your legs and feet. When you stop your muscles should feel soft and relaxed.

Consulting a chiropractor

Having followed the moderate program for two weeks, you should notice a significant improvement in your arthritis; I suggest you now see a chiropractor. During a first visit, the practitioner will observe your posture and how you walk. He or she will then examine your joints as you stand, sit, or lie down, and you will be maneuvered into a number of positions to assess your mobility, flexibility, and nerve function. A chiropractor will use several standard neurological and orthopedic tests when assessing you, and might test your nerve reflexes and, if necessary, request x-rays. During treatment, chiropractors use their hands to help correct misalignments of the spinal vertebrae (called vertebral subluxations). The first treatment session typically lasts 30 to 60 minutes, with follow-up sessions taking 15 to 20 minutes. You might need two or three treatments during the first week, followed by weekly or monthly follow-ups, although this will depend on the exact nature of your problem. To find a chiropractor, check the resources on page 174.

Easy risotto

To make today's risotto, sauté an onion with chopped celery and garlic in olive oil and then add 3¼ cups sliced wild mushrooms. Stir in 1¾ cups risotto rice and add ⅔ cup dry white wine. Slowly stir in 1¼ quarts vegetable stock. When the liquid is absorbed, stir in chopped parsley, a little butter, and some grated Parmesan cheese. Season with freshly ground black pepper.

continuing the moderate program

Well done —you have followed the moderate program for two weeks. You now need to assess whether or not reducing your dietary exposure to nightshade plants has alleviated your arthritis symptoms. Even if you haven't noticed a significant reduction in joint pain and stiffness, I'd still like you to repeat this program so you follow it for a total of 28 days. This is because the glycoalkaloids present in members of the Solanaceae family of plants accumulate in the body, and it can take a month or so for your body to eliminate them.

Your long-term diet

If, after removing nightshade glyocoalkaloids from your diet for four weeks, your symptoms significantly improve, I suggest you continue to avoid members of the nightshade family. To help confirm the link between nightshade plants and arthritis symptoms, consider reintroducing nightshade plants for one day while monitoring your joints closely to see if your symptoms deteriorate. Symptoms produced by glycoalkaloids typically develop after eight to 12 hours, but any flare-up occurring in the one to three days after your trial reintroduction might be a result of nightshade sensitivity. If you're not certain, wait until symptoms settle down, then reintroduce these foods again. Here's a suggested menu plan to reintroduce nightshade plants:

- Breakfast: broiled tomatoes on toast.
- Lunch: tomato soup sprinkled with paprika with one wholewheat bread roll.
- Dinner: Hungarian Goulash (see page 171). Mexican Hot Chili Sauce (see page 169). Boiled, unpeeled potatoes. Tomato salad with chopped red, green, and orange bell peppers.

If eating these foods doesn't trigger a flareup in your symptoms, and you don't feel you have gained significant benefits from the moderate program, then either move back to the gentle program, or try the full-strength program, with its high intake of dietary

Reintroducing potatoes

If you want to eat a normal potato to see if you can tolerate it, make sure it's fresh, and hasn't started to turn even slightly green. Peel it thickly before cooking. Although commercial varieties of potatoes are screened for levels of the glycoalkaloid solanine, most still have a solanine content of up to 0.2 mg/g. Potatoes that are exposed to light and start to turn green, however, can contain solanine concentrations of 1 mg/g or more— mostly in and just under the skin. This is a natural defense to make the potato taste more bitter and, therefore, less likely to be eaten. Potatoes that are damaged during harvesting also produce increased levels of glycoalkaloids, as do those showing signs of disease, such as blight. Eating even a single unpeeled, greening potato can result in a high dose of solanine that can make you feel very ill and upset your joints.

antioxidants to help reduce joint inflammation.If your symptoms *do* worsen after reintroducing nightshade plants, then you have successfully identified the link between your diet and your arthritis symptoms and you should continue to avoid eating tomatoes, potatoes, bell peppers, chilies, eggplants, and related foods. Once you decide to stay on the moderate program long term, continue to follow the principles of the program while taking into account your own likes and dislikes. Always avoid processed, packaged foods, which tend to contain high amounts of the omega-6 essential fatty acids that are converted into inflammatory substances in the body. If you do buy prepared foods, check the labels and avoid foods that contain ingredients such as tomatoes, potato starch, chili, paprika, and so on.

Recipes Explore recipes containing non-nightshade foods, especially healthy, fish-based recipes. You will find some recipe suggestions at www.naturalhealthguru.co.uk and you can post your favorites there, too, for other followers of the moderate program to try.

Your long-term supplement regime

Continue taking the recommended supplements long term. Research supports their use at this moderately high level for significant beneficial effects on joint health. If, up until now, you have taken only the supplements in the recommended list, you might want to add in one or more of the supplements in the optional list for extra benefit. Alternatively, if your arthritis symptoms are well controlled, you might want to reduce the dose of your supplements back down to the levels suggested in the gentle program. If you feel the higher dose suits you better, you can always increase the doses back up to those suggested in the moderate program—or even increase them to those I suggest for the full-strength program.

Your exercise routine

After doing the moderate exercises for four weeks, you should have started to notice an increase in your flexibility. Continue to do the stretch and range-of-motion exercises, ideally twice a day, and fit in the walking or cycling exercise, too (see pages 112–113). Consider starting other activities, such as swimming, dancing, gardening, bowling, or golf—any aerobic activity that you enjoy doing and can do without too much joint discomfort.

You might also want to try the more advanced exercises I show you in the full-strength program—you can start incorporating those into your daily routine, too.

Your therapy program

In the moderate program I have shown you how to use reflexology and other techniques, such as magnetic therapy, homeopathy, herbal medicine, and meditation, which are beneficial for stiff, painful joints. Continue doing these, and keep going to see the natural healthcare professionals—the reflexologist and chiropractor—I suggested, if you found their treatments helpful.

Monitoring your joint symptoms

Keep monitoring and scoring your joint symptoms weekly to make sure you continue to benefit from the moderate program. If your joint scores stop showing an improvement, or start to worsen again, I suggest you increase your supplement doses to those suggested for the full-strength program. Review your diet to see if you ate any nightshade plants that might have triggered your symptoms. If not, it's possible you have developed a sensitivity to another food. Consult a naturopath or a nutritionist with training in the field of food intolerances. Continue to eat a balanced diet while still avoiding your individual trigger foods.

breakfast recipes

green tea compote

serves 4

8 semidried apricots, pitted and
    chopped
8 semidried prunes, pitted and chopped
8 dates, pitted and chopped
8 dried figs, chopped
1 handful raisins
3 cups hot green tea
1 handful pistachio nuts
Lowfat fromage blanc or plain yogurt
    with live cultures, to serve

1 Place the fruit in an heatproof
   bowl, pour the green tea over,
   and leave to steep until cold, or
   overnight in the refrigerator.

2 Sprinkle with pistachio nuts
   and serve with fromage blanc
   or yogurt.

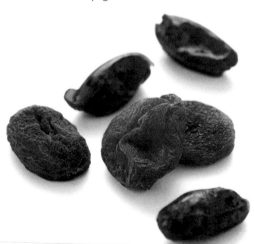

apple, kiwi, and watercress smoothie

serves 4

4 red eating apples, cored
4 kiwifruit, peeled
1 handful of watercress
Scant ½ cup unsweetened apple juice

1 Whiz all the ingredients
   together in a blender.

2 Add more apple juice if you
   prefer a lighter smoothie.

fresh figs with blueberries

serves 4

8 fresh figs
4 handfuls blueberries
½ cup lowfat fromage blanc or plain
    yogurt with live cultures

1 Make two deep crosses in the
   tops of the figs, then gently
   open them into a "tulip" shape.

2 Mix the blueberries with the
   fromage blanc or yogurt, saving
   a few blueberries for garnish.

3 Spoon the berry mixture into
   the figs, with the remainder on
   the side. Sprinkle the reserved
   berries over the top.

omega-3 omelet with smoked trout and tarragon

serves 4

2 tablespoons olive oil
8 omega-3-enriched eggs, lightly beaten
5 ounces smoked trout fillet, skinned
    and flaked
1 handful chopped tarragon
Freshly ground black pepper

1 Heat the olive oil in a large
   nonstick skillet over high heat.
   Tip in the eggs and gather the
   curds into the middle as the
   egg sets, so more runny egg
   covers the pan.

2 As soon as there's only a little
   runny egg left, remove the pan
   from the heat. Scatter the trout
   and tarragon over one half of
   the omelet and season with
   black pepper.

3 Return to the heat and warm
   through for 30 seconds. Fold
   the omelet in half, slide out
   onto a plate and serve.

lunch recipes

herring with oats and pecans

serves 4

. . . .

2 handfuls Scotch oats
2 handfuls pecan nuts, finely chopped
4 small herring, cleaned and scaled with
 backbones removed
4 tablespoons lowfat or nonfat milk
2 tablespoons olive oil
Grated zest and juice of 1 unwaxed
 lemon
1 bunch watercress
Freshly ground black pepper

1 Mix together the oats and
 pecans in a bowl.
2 Dip the herrings in the milk,
 then roll them in the oat
 and pecan mixture until
 evenly coated. Season with
 black pepper.
3 Heat the olive oil in a skillet and
 fry the herring over low heat 10
 minutes on each side. Sprinkle
 each fish with the lemon zest
 and juice, then serve on a bed
 of watercress.

tuna, pomegranate, and anchovy salad

serves 4

. . . .

2 cans (6-oz.) tuna flakes in olive oil,
 drained
4 handfuls mixed salad leaves
1 handful watercress
1 bulb fennel, chopped
1 pomegranate, seeds removed (see
 page 102)
4 anchovy fillets in oil, drained
Ciabatta bread, sliced, to serve

For the dressing:
3 anchovy fillets in oil, drained
1 garlic clove, crushed
¾ cup crème fraîche or sour cream
Grated zest and juice of 1 unwaxed
 lemon
Freshly ground black pepper

1 Whiz all the dressing
 ingredients in a blender and
 season with black pepper.
2 Mix all the salad ingredients
 together except the anchovies.
 Pour the dressing over the top.
 Sprinkle with the anchovies and
 serve with ciabatta.

avocado and smoked salmon oriental salad

serves 4

. . . .

4½ ounces rice noodles
1 red onion, finely chopped
½ cucumber, chopped
1 avocado, halved, pitted, and peeled
3 ounces smoked salmon, cut in strips
1 handful mixed baby salad leaves
1 handful toasted sesame seeds

For the dressing:
4 tablespoons walnut oil
1 garlic clove, crushed
1 tablespoon red wine vinegar
1 tablespoon chopped cilantro leaves
Freshly ground black pepper

1 Cook the noodles (follow the
 package directions) and drain.
2 Put the dressing ingredients in
 a screw-top jar and shake well.
3 Mix all the salad ingredients
 together, then toss them in
 the salad dressing and serve.

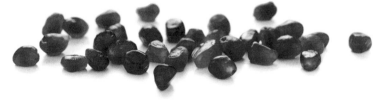

spicy sweet potato salad

· ·

serves 4

2 tablespoons extra virgin olive oil
1 garlic clove, crushed
1 teaspoon cumin seeds
1 teaspoon coriander seeds
2 large, orange-red sweet potatoes,
    peeled and cubed
1 can (15-oz.) chickpeas, drained
1 red onion, chopped
2½ cups baby spinach leaves
1 handful cilantro leaves
1 handful pumpkin seeds

For the dressing:
7 tablespoons lowfat plain yogurt with
    live cultures
Grated zest and juice of 1 orange
Freshly ground black pepper

1 Heat the oven to 400°F.
2 Mix the olive oil, garlic, cumin, and coriander seeds in a large bowl. Toss the sweet potatoes in the spicy oil.
3 Roast the sweet potatoes 20 minutes, or until tender; set aside to cool. Mix the dressing ingredients together and season with black pepper.
4 Mix the cold sweet potatoes with the remaining salad ingredients and drizzle with the yogurt dressing.

pear, avocado, and blue cheese salad

· ·

serves 4

2 dessert pears, quartered, cored, and
    sliced
2 avocados, halved, pitted, and peeled
Grated zest and juice of 2 lemons
4 handfuls mixed salad leaves
3 ounces blue cheese, such as
    dolcelatte, gorgonzola, Roquefort, or
    Stilton, crumbled
½ cup pecans, chopped
4 tablespoons walnut oil

1 Mix the pears and avocados with the lemon zest and juice.
2 Put a handful of salad leaves on each of four plates. Pile the pear mixture on top and sprinkle with the blue cheese and the pecans. Drizzle with walnut oil and serve.

lentil, sweet potato, and apricot soup

serves 4

2 tablespoons extra virgin olive oil
1 red onion, chopped
2 garlic cloves, crushed
1 teaspoon cumin seeds, freshly ground
1 tablespoon coriander seeds, freshly ground
½ cup red lentils
²/₃ cup semidried apricots
1 sweet potato, peeled and diced
2 carrots, peeled and grated
Grated zest and juice of 1 unwaxed lemon
1 quart vegetable stock or water
²/₃ cup lowfat plain yogurt with live cultures
1 handful cilantro leaves, chopped
Freshly ground black pepper

1 Heat the olive oil in a pan and sauté the onion, garlic, cumin, and coriander seeds until the onion starts to color. Add all the remaining soup ingredients, except the yogurt and cilantro, and bring to a boil.

2 Cover and simmer 30 minutes. Puree in a blender until smooth. Season to taste with black pepper, add a swirl of yogurt, and serve sprinkled with cilantro leaves.

left: spicy sweet potato salad

dinner recipes

herby pecan nut roast

serves 4

1 large onion, chopped
2 garlic cloves, chopped
2 tablespoons extra virgin olive oil

For the herb mix ture:
1 handful mixed herbs, such as parsley, thyme, marjoram, and sage, chopped
1¼ cups fresh wholewheat bread crumbs
1 omega-3-enriched egg, beaten
Freshly ground black pepper

For the nut mixture:
1½ cups pecans, finely chopped
1½ cups fresh wholewheat bread crumbs
²/₃ cup vegetable stock or water
Grated zest and juice of 1 unwaxed lemon
Freshly ground black pepper

1 Heat the oven to 400°F.

2 Line an 8- x 4-inch bread pan with wax paper. Heat the oil in a pan and fry the onion and garlic. Divide the mixture in half. Mix one half with the herb mixture ingredients; set aside.

3 Add the remaining onion to the nut mixture ingredients. Put half the nut mix into the bread pan. Add the herb mixture, then the remaining nut mixture.

4 Bake 30 minutes, or until lightly brown. Leave to cool slightly, then turn out and serve.

braised red cabbage with apple and red wine

serves 4

1 red cabbage, shredded
1 red onion, chopped
2 Red Delicious apples, cored and chopped
½ cup red wine
2 tablespoons red wine vinegar
3 tablespoons dark brown sugar
3 cloves
2 cinnamon sticks
¼ teaspoon grated nutmeg
2 tablespoons butter
Freshly ground black pepper

1 Heat the oven to 300°F.

2 Mix all the ingredients in a baking dish with an ovenproof cover. Cover and bake 3 hours, stirring every 30 minutes.

smoked haddock omelet with béchamel sauce

serves 4

2 cups lowfat or nonfat milk
1 clove
1 bay leaf
1 onion, chopped
7 ounces undyed smoked haddock, flaked
8 omega-3-enriched eggs, beaten
2 tablespoons butter
¼ cup all-purpose flour
2 tablespoons extra virgin olive oil
1 cup grated Parmesan
1 handful parsley, finely chopped
Freshly ground black pepper

1 Bring the milk, clove, bay leaf, and onion to a boil in a small pan. Add the haddock and simmer slowly until the fish is tender; remove from the heat.
2 Strain the milk mixture and discard the clove. Melt the butter in a pan, sprinkle the flour over and stir in. Slowly add the strained milk and whisk to create a smooth sauce.
3 Heat the olive oil in a pan and cook the egg until it is just set.
4 Add the flaked haddock and spoon the béchamel sauce over. Sprinkle the Parmesan on top and and place under a hot broiler until bubbling. Sprinkle with parsley, season with black pepper, and serve hot.

oaty mackerel with beet salsa

serves 4

4 mackerel fillets
Olive oil for brushing
1 handful oatmeal
Freshly ground black pepper

For the salsa:
2 beets
1 red onion, finely sliced
¼ cucumber, peeled and diced
2 celery sticks, finely chopped
1 carrot, peeled and grated
Grated zest and juice of 1 unwaxed lemon
4 tablespoons extra virgin olive oil
1 handful herbs, such as parsley, chives, and cilantro, chopped

1 Heat the oven to 400°F.
2 Boil the beets (unpeeled) in water 30 minutes, or until cooked. Drain and leave to cool, then peel and dice.
3 Mix all the salsa ingredients and leave to infuse.
4 Brush the mackerel with olive oil and dip in the oatmeal to coat evenly; season well with black pepper.
5 Put the fillets on a baking tray and bake 10 minutes, or until cooked though. Leave to cool and serve warm with the salsa.

marinated herring

serves 4

4 herring fillets, skinned and cut into bite-size pieces

For the marinade:
1 cup dry white wine
2 tablespoons white wine vinegar
1 teaspoon honey
1 large scallion, finely chopped
1 bay leaf
6 peppercorns, green, red, and black mixed, crushed
1 handful dill, chopped

For the dressing:
$2/3$ cup lowfat plain yogurt with live cultures
2 tablespoons wholegrain mustard
4 tablespoons chopped dill
2 teaspoons honey
Grated zest and juice of 1 unwaxed lemon
Freshly ground black pepper

1 Put all the marinade ingredients in a pan. Cover and simmer slowly 15 minutes.
2 Put the herring fillets in a shallow, nonmetallic dish and pour the boiling marinade over them; cover and leave to cool.
3 Mix the dressing ingredients together and season to taste.
4 Remove the herring from the marinade (and discard the marinade). Mix the herring with the yogurt dressing and serve chilled.

macadamia nut and lemon juice dressing

serves 4

4 tablespoons macadamia nut oil
Grated zest and juice of 1 large
    unwaxed lemon
Freshly ground black pepper

1 Put the ingredients in a
    screwtop jar and shake well.

baked whole fish with lemon and herbs

serves 4

1 whole round fish, about 3 pounds
    5 ounces, such as sea bass, trout, or
    salmon, dressed, scaled, and rinsed
    inside and out
2 tablespoons extra virgin olive oil, or
    herb-flavored olive oil
1 handful mixed herbs, such as fennel,
    dill, thyme, and rosemary
1 handful parsley, chopped
1 unwaxed lemon, sliced
Freshly ground black pepper

1 Heat the oven to 375°F.
2 Brush the fish inside and
    out with the olive oil and
    season with black pepper. Fill
    the body of the fish with the
    herbs and put the lemon slices
    on the outside of the fish.
3 Wrap the fish in greased foil
    and bake 30 to 45 minutes until
    it is cooked through and the
    flesh flakes easily when tested
    with a knife.

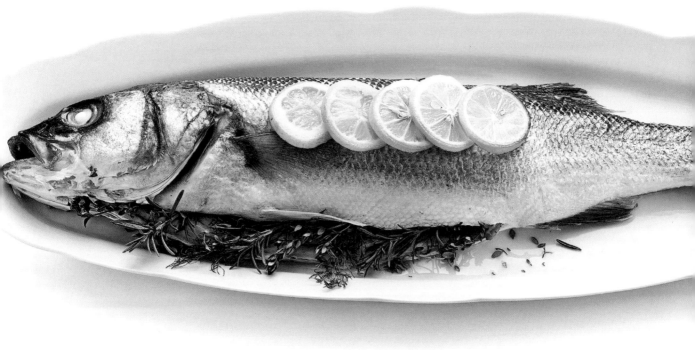

baked whole fish with lemon and herbs

delicious black beans

serves 4

2 tablespoon olive oil
1 large onion, chopped
2 garlic cloves, crushed
2 celery sticks, finely chopped
1 large carrot, peeled and grated
1 handful mixed herbs, such as parsley,
    oregano, and basil, chopped
1 pinch ground cloves
1 heaped cup dried black beans,
    washed and soaked overnight with
    the liquid reserved
1 bouillon cube (beef, chicken or
    vegetable)
1 bay leaf
2 teaspoon red wine vinegar
Freshly ground black pepper

1 Heat the olive oil in a pan and
   sauté the onion, garlic, celery,
   carrot, herbs, and ground
   cloves until the onion starts
   to brown.

2 Add the beans to the onion
   mixture together with enough
   of the soaking liquid to cover
   the ingredients by at least
   2 inches.

3 Add the bouillon cube and bay
   leaf and bring to a boil. Cover
   and simmer 2 hours, stirring
   occasionally. Stir in the vinegar
   and season well with black
   pepper. Continue cooking 30
   minutes longer, or until the
   beans are tender. Remove the
   bay leaf and serve.

pesto sauce

serves 4

1 cup firmly packed basil leaves
½ cup pecans, chopped
3 garlic cloves, crushed
¾ cup extra virgin olive oil
1 handful freshly grated Parmesan
    cheese
1 handful freshly grated pecorino
    cheese, or more Parmesan
Freshly ground black pepper

1 Whiz all the ingredients in a
   blender until smooth. Or, if you
   prefer a coarser texture, grind
   each ingredient in turn using
   a pestle and mortar, then add
   the olive oil a little at a time.

2 Season with black pepper
   to taste.

pesto and tuna ciabatta pizzas

serves 4

2 part-baked ciabatta, halved lengthwise
1 recipe quantity Pesto Sauce (see
    previous recipe)
1 can (6½oz.) tuna in olive oil, flaked
    and drained
1 handful black olives, pitted and halved
4 handfuls grated cheese (cheddar or
    mozzarella)
Freshly ground black pepper

1 Heat the oven to 350°F.

2 Spread each half of the
   ciabattas with pesto and
   place cut-side up on a baking

sheet. Sprinkle each one with
a quarter of the flaked tuna,
olives, and cheese. Bake 20
minutes.

pasta with walnuts and cilantro

serves 4

6 tablespoons walnut oil
4 handfuls walnuts, chopped
2 garlic cloves, crushed
1 teaspoon coriander seeds, crushed
1 handful cilantro leaves, chopped
1 pound fresh pasta, or 12 ounces dried
    pasta
⅔ cup grated Parmesan
Freshly ground black pepper

1 Blend or pound the walnut
   oil, walnuts, garlic, coriander
   seeds, and cilantro leaves into
   a smooth paste. Season with
   black pepper.

2 Cook the pasta in plenty of
   boiling water until al dente.
   Drain but leave moist so the
   sauce coats the pasta well.

3 Mix the pasta with the walnut
   and cilantro mixture, toss well
   and sprinkle with Parmesan.
   Leave to marinate for at least 1
   hour, then reheat and serve.

pasta with smoked salmon and fennel

serves 4

2 tablespoons olive oil
2 garlic cloves, crushed
1 onion, chopped
1 small bulb fennel, chopped into
  matchsticks, with the green fronds
  reserved
Grated zest and juice of 1 unwaxed
  lemon
1¼ cups Greek yogurt
7 ounces smoked salmon, chopped
1 pound fresh wholewheat pasta, or 12
  ounces dried pasta
Freshly ground black pepper

1 Heat the olive oil in a pan and
   sauté the garlic, onion, and
   chopped fennel until starting to
   color. Add the lemon zest and
   juice and yogurt. Heat through,
   stirring continuously. Don't boil
   or the yogurt might curdle.
2 Remove from the heat and
   stir in the smoked salmon.
   Meanwhile, cook the pasta in
   plenty of boiling water until al
   dente. Drain, but leave moist
   so the sauce will coats the
   pasta well. Combine the pasta
   and sauce. Season with some
   black pepper.
3 Toss well, sprinkle the chopped
   fennel fronds on top, and serve.

dessert recipes

baked apples with cloves

serves 4

⅓ cup semidried apricots, chopped
3 cups hot black, green, or white tea
4 cooking apples, cored
16 cloves
½ cup raisins
4 tablespoons butter
¼ cup firmly packed soft brown sugar

1 Heat the oven to 350°F.
2 Soak the apricots in hot tea
   10 minutes. Meanwhile, peel
   the top quarter of each apple
   and stud the flesh with
   4 cloves. Place in a baking dish.
3 Mix the soaked apricots with
   the raisins, butter, and sugar.
   Use the mixture to fill the cored
   middle of each apple. Pour
   a little hot tea in the dish with
   the apples to a depth of about
   ⅛ inch.
4 Bake 45 minutes until the
   apples are soft. Remove the
   cloves and serve with the juice
   from the pan.

raspberry and red wine sorbet

serves 4

2 heaped cups raspberries, fresh or
  thawed from frozen
7 ounces light red wine, such as
  Beaujolais or Valpolicella
¼ cup sugar

1 Put all the ingredients in a
   pan, stirring until the sugar
   dissolves, then bring to a boil.
   Simmer 5 minutes, without
   stirring.
2 Cool and put in the freezer at
   least 3 hours, churning up the
   ice crystals occasionally.

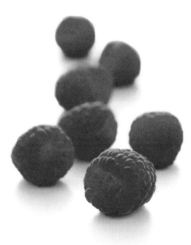

cinnamon-chocolate nut terrine

• •

serves 8

Oil for brushing the pan
14 ounces bittersweet chocolate (at
    least 70 percent cocoa solids)
1¼ cups heavy cream
2 teaspoons ground cinnamon
1 tablespoon sugar
3½ cups pecans, halved

1　Lightly brush an 8½- x 4-inch
    bread pan with the oil, and line
    with plastic wrap, leaving some
    overhanging. Partially melt the
    chocolate in a bowl over a pan
    of hot water. In a separate pan,
    heat the cream to just below
    boiling point.
2　Remove the partially melted
    chocolate from the heat and
    add the hot cream, stirring until
    the chocolate fully melts.
3　Stir in the cinnamon and sugar.
    Place a layer of pecans in the
    bottom of the bread pan, then
    pour some of the chocolate
    mixture over. Keep layering,
    finishing with chocolate. Chill
    at least 2 hours, then remove
    from the pan, discard the
    plastic wrap, and serve.

chocolate lava pudding

• •

serves 6

1¾ sticks unsalted butter, softened, with
    the butter paper resreved
½ cup all-purpose flour, plus extra for
    dusting
10 ounces bittersweet chocolate (at
    least 70 percent cocoa solids)
²⁄₃ cup soft light brown sugar sugar
4 omega-3-enriched eggs, beaten
1 teaspoon vanilla extract

1　Heat the oven to 400°F.
2　Use the butter paper to grease
    6 ramekins, then dust them
    with flour. Melt the chocolate
    on a plate over a pan of
    hot water.
3　Cream together the butter and
    sugar, then beat in the eggs
    and vanilla extract. Add the
    flour to make a smooth batter,
    then stir in the chocolate.
4　Divide the batter between the
    ramekins and bake 10 minutes;
    serve hot.

berry and hazelnut meringue

• •

serves 4

4 omega-3-enriched eggs, whites only
¾ cup plus 1 tablespoon superfine
    sugar
1 cup lowfat fromage blanc or plain
    yogurt with live cultures
10 ounces berries, such as strawberries,
    raspberries, blueberries, or
    blackberries
¾ cup skinned hazelnuts, toasted and
    chopped
1 small handful chopped mint leaves

1　Heat the oven to 275°F.
2　Beat the egg whites until they
    form stiff peaks. Gradually beat
    in the sugar to form a glossy,
    thick, white meringue. Spread
    the meringue in a rough 9-inch
    circle on a sheet of baking
    parchment.
3　Bake in the oven about
    1 hour, or until the meringue is
    crisp on the outside; remove
    and leave to cool.
4　Spread the fromage frais or
    yogurt over the meringue and
    sprinkle the berries, toasted
    hazelnuts, and mint over
    the top.

right: berry and hazelnut meringue

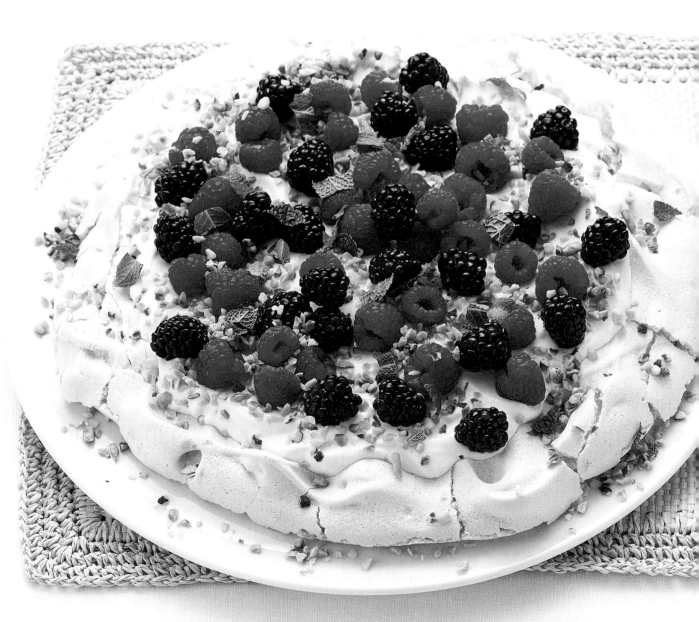

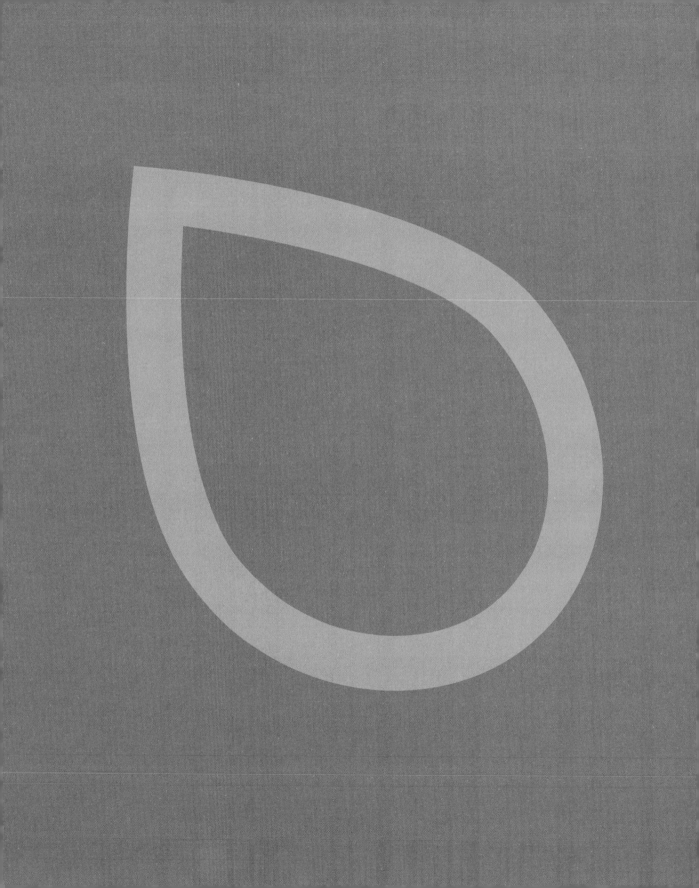

introducing the full-strength program

The full-strength program is ideal for people whose arthritis symptoms didn't significantly improve while following the Mediterranean-style diet of the gentle program or the exclusion diet of the moderate program. I also recommend it if your arthritis is associated with the inflammation (red, swollen joints) that's common in rheumatoid and other autoimmune forms of arthritis.

The full-strength program diet

The full-strength program offers a way to eat that is exceptionally high in antioxidants. It incorporates foods with a high Oxygen Radical Absorbance Capacity (ORAC; see pages 47–49) value, such as bittersweet chocolate, blueberries, red kidney beans, cranberries, Red Delicious apples, Russet potatoes, and plums —these typically provide more than 4,000 ORAC units per average serving. Some of the other arthritis superfoods in the program offer fewer ORAC units, but I've made sure they each provide more than 1,000 ORAC units per average serving—they soon add up.

The average person eating a typical Western diet obtains an estimated 5,700 ORAC units a day. Ideally, you need to obtain at least 7,000 ORAC units a day for good health. The full-strength program offers you at least 20,000 ORAC units per day from diet alone. This has the potential to significantly reduce inflammation linked to free-radical damage within your joints.

Eating lots of chilies The full-strength program diet includes chilies and other spices, which, as well as having an antioxidant potential, also have a medicinal, analgesic action in the body. Chili peppers contain natural analgesic compounds known as capsaicinoids and are particularly beneficial for arthritis—as long as you're not sensitive to the nightshade family of plants (see page 51). As the full-strength program also includes other members of the nightshade family —potatoes, tomatoes, bell peppers, and eggplants— you need to be sure eating them doesn't worsen your arthritis. If you're unsure, go back and complete the moderate program to find out.

Capsaicinoids, such as capsaicin, dihydrocapsaicin, nordihydrocapsaicin, homodihydrocapsaicin, and homocapsaicin, are irritants found in the flesh of chili peppers, which are especially concentrated in the white tissue supporting the seeds. As well as producing the burning sensations that occur when you eat chilies, capsaicinoids have painkilling properties. They overwhelm pain-detecting nerves and prevent them from passing on additional pain messages. Capsaicin also blocks the activity of decapeptide substance P (DSP), thereby protecting against cartilage breakdown in osteoarthritis.

The capsaicin content and hotness of chili peppers is measured according to the Scoville scale (see page 159), in which a sweet bell pepper has a Scoville rating of zero (no capsaicin), while the hottest chili, the habanero, has a rating of 200,000 plus, which means its juice must be diluted more than 200,000 times before the capsaicin becomes undetectable. The hotter the pepper, the higher the capsaicin content and the more potentially beneficial it is for arthritis pain.

Shopping list

Base your shopping lists on the following items, which feature in the menu plans and recipes. Buy regularly in small quantities.

drinks
apple juice (unsweetened), blueberry juice, cranberry juice, mineral water (low sodium), pomegranate juice, red wine (Beaujolais), and herbal, fruit, and green, black, or white tea

dairy products
butter (unsalted), crème fraîche fromage blanc (plain), milk (lowfat and nonfat); lowfat vanilla ice cream; yogurt (vanilla and plain lowfat with live cultures); cheeses: cottage cheese, cheddar, feta, Gruyère, mozzarella, Parmesan

fruit
apples (Red Delicious and cooking apples), bananas, blackberries, blueberries, cherries, cranberries (dried and fresh), dates, figs (dried and fresh), grapes (black), kiwifruit, lemons, limes, mangoes, oranges, peaches, plums, prunes, raisins, raspberries, strawberries

vegetables
avocados, beets, bell peppers (red, green, yellow), black beans, broccoli, cabbage (red), carrots, celery, chickpeas, corn, cucumber, eggplants, Florence fennel, globe artichoke, green beans, kale, kidney beans (dried), lentils (red), lettuce (red oak leaf, lollo rosso, hearts), mixed red salad leaves, onions (red), peas, purple sprouting broccoli, red kidney beans, Russet potatoes, spinach, sweet potatoes, tomatoes (regular and beefsteak), zucchini

nuts and seeds
almonds, mixed seeds, pecans, pistachios, walnuts

herbs, spices, oils and vinegar
basil, bay leaf, black pepper, cardamom pods, cayenne pepper, chilies (red, green), cilantro, cinnamon (ground and sticks), cloves, coriander (ground and seeds), cumin, dill, fenugreek, garlic, ginger, mustard seeds, oregano/marjoram, paprika (hot and sweet), parsley, peppercorns (black, pink), saffron, turmeric; extra virgin and standard olive oil, pecan oil, walnut oil; red wine vinegar, rice wine vinegar

grains
bulgur wheat, high-fiber breakfast cereals, noodles, old-fashioned rolled oats, rice (basmati, brown, long-grain, and red), speciality breads (ciabatta, focaccia, sun-dried tomato, garlic and herb), wholewheat/multigrain bread and rolls, wholewheat flour (plain, self-rising), wholewheat pita bread

proteins
omega-3-enriched eggs; seafood: mackerel (smoked), salmon (fresh and smoked), shrimp, tuna (fresh or in olive oil), white fish (for example, bream, red snapper, or sea bass); meat: beef (tenderloin), boneless, skinless chicken breast halves, ham, stewing steak

miscellaneous
baking powder, bean salad (canned), black bean sauce (organic), coconut milk, shredded coconut, bittersweet chocolate (at least 70 percent cocoa solids), dried skim milk powder, powdered gelatin (unflavored), honey, maple syrup, mayonnaise (low fat), wholegarin mustard, olive-oil spread, red pesto sauce, tomato paste, bouillon cubes (vegetable), sugar (Demerara, confectioners', and granulated), tortilla chips, vanilla bean or extract

Eating other arthritis superfoods The full-strength diet features red lentils, which are one of the richest plant sources of protein and which also have an unusually high ORAC score. It also includes beets —a source of unique pigments called betalains, such as betanin, which, as well as giving beets their dark, attractive color and earthy flavor, have a powerful antioxidant action.

For your daily snacks, I have suggested high-ORAC-score fruits, such as berries and Red Delicious apples. During this program, your daily nut snack consists of either pecans or walnuts, which, as well as having an excellent antioxidant content, are good sources of anti-inflammatory omega-3 fatty acids.

Losing weight Although it's not designed for weight loss, you should find that you lose any excess weight slowly and naturally while following this healthy-eating program. If you want to speed up the process of weight loss, eat smaller portions, especially of the starchy foods, such as pasta, bread and rice, and replace dessert recipes with high-ORAC fruits.

The full-strength program exercise routine

Your exercise routine involves a series of stretches that will help improve joint flexibility. Repeat these once or twice a day, adding each day's exercise to the previous one(s). In addition, you should aim to do regular brisk aerobic exercise. Use heat and ice, as explained on page 31, to help prepare your joints for exercise, and to treat them afterward if necessary.

Walking, cycling, and swimming are all good choices of aerobic exercise. Swimming builds strength, stamina, and suppleness and is especially good for weight-bearing joints, such as your back, hips, knees, and ankles. Here's a suggested regime to help you slowly increase the amount of exercise you do over a

Full-strength program supplements

These are the supplements that I feel are the most beneficial on the full-strength program. Read about them on pages 58–63 to help you decide which you want to take. You can, of course, take all of them, as I have designed this plan to include supplements with the best synergistic action. Supplements are widely available from drug stores, supermarkets, and healthfood stores.

recommended daily supplements

- Glucosamine sulfate (1,500 mg)
- Chondroitin (1,200 mcg)
- MSM (1 g)
- Vitamin C (1,000 mg, twice daily)
- Omega-3 fish oils (900 mg daily, for example, 3 x 1-g fish oil capsules, each supplying 180 mg EPA + 120 mg DHA)
- Evening primrose oil (2,000 mg)

optional daily supplements (these provide additional benefits)

- Vitamin-B complex (75 mg)
- Vitamin D (15 mcg)
- Vitamin E (400 mg/600 iu)
- Calcium (800 mg)
- Selenium (200 mcg)
- Green-lipped mussel extracts—especially for inflammatory forms of arthritis such as rheumatoid (600–900 mg)
- Garlic tablets—especially if you have rheumatoid arthritis (allicin yield 1,500 mcg)

two-month period (assuming that you stay on the full-strength program). Remember to warm up and cool down first.

- Week one: walk, cycle, or swim for 20 minutes on Tuesday, Thursday, and Saturday.
- Week two: walk, cycle, or swim for 20 minutes on Tuesday and Saturday, and for 25 minutes on Thursday.
- Week three: walk, cycle, or swim for 20 minutes on Thursday and Sunday, and for 25 minutes on Tuesday and Saturday.
- Week four: walk, cycle, or swim for 25 minutes on Tuesday, Thursday, Saturday, and Sunday.
- Week five: walk, cycle, or swim for 25 minutes on Thursday and Sunday, and for 30 minutes on Tuesday and Saturday.
- Week six: walk, cycle or swim for 30 minutes on Tuesday, Thursday, Saturday, and Sunday.
- Week seven: walk, cycle, or swim for 30 minutes on Thursday and Sunday, and for 35 minutes on Tuesday and Saturday.
- Week eight: walk, cycle, or swim for 35 minutes on Tuesday and Saturday, and for 40 minutes on Thursday and Sunday.

The full-strength program therapies

During this program, I show you some acupressure techniques to do at home, followed by other holistic approaches. I suggest that you book an appointment with an acupuncturist and a Reiki practitioner now in preparation for days seven and fourteen.

the full-strength program day one

Daily menu

- **Breakfast: Toast with Berry and Apple Jelly (see page 165)**

- **Morning snack: Red Delicious apple or a handful of black grapes**

- **Lunch: globe artichoke with chopped dates, figs, tomatoes, basil, and mozzarella cheese. Mixed red salad leaves drizzled with Pecan Oil and Red Wine Vinegar Dressing (see page 168). Pita bread. "High-ORAC" fruit (see page 49)**

- **Afternoon snack: handful of pecans**

- **Dinner: Extra-Spicy Chili Beans (see page 172). Red rice. Mashed avocado with lemon juice. Mixed red salad leaves drizzled with Pecan Oil and Red Wine Vinegar Dressing (see page 168). About 1½ ounces bittersweet chocolate. A handful of cherries**

- **Drinks: 2½ cups lowfat or nonfat milk. Unlimited tea (including herbal or fruit tea) and mineral water. Glass of pomegranate, blueberry, cranberry, or apple juice**

- **Supplements: see page 145**

Your dinner tonight is extra-spicy chili beans. If you have a good tolerance for spicy food, add some Mexican hot chili sauce—the analgesic compounds in chilies are good for your joints.

Daily exercise routine

The exercises I show you over the following two weeks are stretches that will help strengthen your muscles and maintain your joint flexibility. They will help you to stay active and mobile. Repeat them once or twice a day, adding each day's exercise to the one(s) you've learned previously. You should also start your walking, cycling, or swimming regime, as described on pages 144–145.

Forward stretches

1 Stand comfortably, feet slightly apart, arms by your sides. Bend forward as if to touch your toes.

2 Stretch down with your arms and fingers as far down your legs as is comfortable.

3 Maintain your maximum stretch for five seconds. Flex your knees slightly and put your hands on your knees to help you stand up. Stand straight with your shoulders back and relax before repeating the stretch at least once more.

Acupressure

During this first week, I'm going to show you how to use acupressure to reduce joint pain. Today's acupressure point is Large Intestine 4, also known as LI4, *HeGu*, or Union Valley—don't use this point if you are pregnant.

Large Intestine 4

1 LI4 is on the back of your hand in the web between your thumb and index finger. To find it, bring your thumb and index finger close together and feel around the highest spot of the muscle bulge that forms from the web on the back of your hand—the point is likely to feel tender. Start by pressing lightly, and gradually increase the pressure to the limit of comfort.

2 Release the pressure gradually and then build it up. Press for one minute while breathing slowly and deeply. If your joint pains are worse on your left side, use LI4 on your right hand for relief, and vice versa.

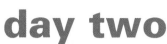

day two

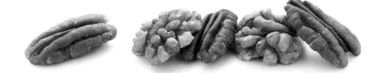

Daily menu

- **Breakfast: Apple and Carrot Breakfast Muffins (see page 164)**

- **Morning snack: Red Delicious apple or a handful of black grapes**

- **Lunch: Borscht Soup (see page 166). Wholewheat bread roll. "High-ORAC" fruit (see page 49)**

- **Afternoon snack: handful of walnuts**

- **Dinner: poached or steamed fish fillet. Spinach. Carrots drizzled with plain lowfat yogurt with live cultures. Mashed potato made with Russet potatoes. Chocolate, Prune, and Pecan Squares (see page 173)**

- **Drinks: 2½ cups lowfat or nonfat milk. Unlimited tea (including herbal or fruit tea) and mineral water. Glass of pomegranate, blueberry, cranberry, or apple juice**

- **Supplements: see page 145**

Daily exercise routine

Continue with the walking, cycling, or swimming regime suggested on pages 144–145. Do yesterday's forward stretch, then these side bends. If today's exercise, or any other exercise, makes you feel dizzy, unstable, or uncomfortable, stop straightaway—see the caution about knowing your limits on page 115.

Side bends

1 Stand comfortably with your feet apart and your hands by your sides. Slowly bend sideways to your left, so your left hand travels down your leg as far as is comfortable.

2 Slowly straighten and repeat on the right side. (Take care not to lean forward or backward as you bend.) Repeat so you do five bends to the left and five to the right.

3 To make this exercise easier, modify it by flexing your knees slightly and walking your hands up your legs when you stand up from a bend. You can also stabilize yourself by doing the exercise with your back against a wall.

Acupressure

Work on yesterday's acupressure point and then today's: Governing Vessel 14, also known as DU14, *DaZhui*, or the Great Hammer. This point is used in Chinese medicine to strengthen the neck and spine, and to dispel the invasion of wind and cold, which in Chinese medicine is believed to be responsible for causing painful muscles and joints.

Governing vessel 14

1 This point is located between your seventh cervical (neck) vertebra and the spinous process of your first thoracic vertebra, approximately level with your shoulders. To find it, bend your head forward and run a finger down the back of your neck. Find the most prominent bone and then feel for the hollow just beneath—it can feel slightly tender.

2 Stimulate the point by slowly increasing the pressure to the limit of comfort and then gradually releasing it. Keep pressing in this way for one minute while breathing slowly and deeply.

the full-strength program day three

Daily menu

- **Breakfast: Omelet with Caramelized Sweet Potato and Red Onions (see page 165). Wilted baby spinach. Sliced tomatoes**

- **Morning snack: Red Delicious apple or a handful of black grapes**

- **Lunch: smoked mackerel. Shredded red cabbage, carrot, beet, and red onion. Mixed red salad leaves with Pecan Oil and Red Wine Vinegar Dressing (see page 168). Specialty bread. "High-ORAC" fruit (see page 49)**

- **Afternoon snack: handful of pecans**

- **Dinner: Hungarian Goulash (see page 171). Red or brown rice. Mixed red salad leaves with Pecan Oil and Red Wine Vinegar Dressing (see page 168). Vanilla ice cream with Fresh Strawberry Coulis (see page 172)**

- **Drinks: 2½ cups lowfat or nonfat milk. Unlimited tea (including herbal or fruit tea) and mineral water. Glass of pomegranate, blueberry, cranberry, or apple juice**

- **Supplements: see page 145**

Daily exercise routine

Walk, cycle, or swim (see pages 144–145) and do the stretch exercises from days one and two, followed by these wall presses.

Wall presses

1 Stand facing a wall with your feet hip-width apart, your back straight, your abdominal muscles pulled in, and your pelvis tilted forward. Place your hands flat on the wall in line with your shoulders.

2 Do wall presses by bending your elbows and leaning in so your nose almost touches the wall—keep your back flat and your legs straight. Hold this position briefly, then use your arms to push away from the wall. Breathe in as you lean in; breathe out as you push out. Repeat five to 10 times.

Acupressure

Work on the sequence of acupressure points you have learned so far, then stimulate Bladder 11, also known as BI11, *DaShu*, or Great Shuttle point. This will disperse wind from your joints and bones.

Bladder 11

1 Locate the point two finger widths away from the spine on each side, below the Great Hammer (see page 147) and level with the space between your first and second thoracic vertebrae.

2 Stimulate BI11 on your left side by putting your right hand over your left shoulder, and vice versa. Stimulate as usual by slowly increasing pressure, then releasing it over a period of a minute while breathing slowly and deeply.

Red wine

If you would like the occasional glass of red wine, feel free to indulge (but don't have more than two or three a week). The antioxidant activity of one glass (5 ounces) of red wine is equivalent to that of 12 glasses white wine. Watch out for any flareup in your arthritis symptoms a day or two after drinking wine though, because some people have an alcohol intolerance.

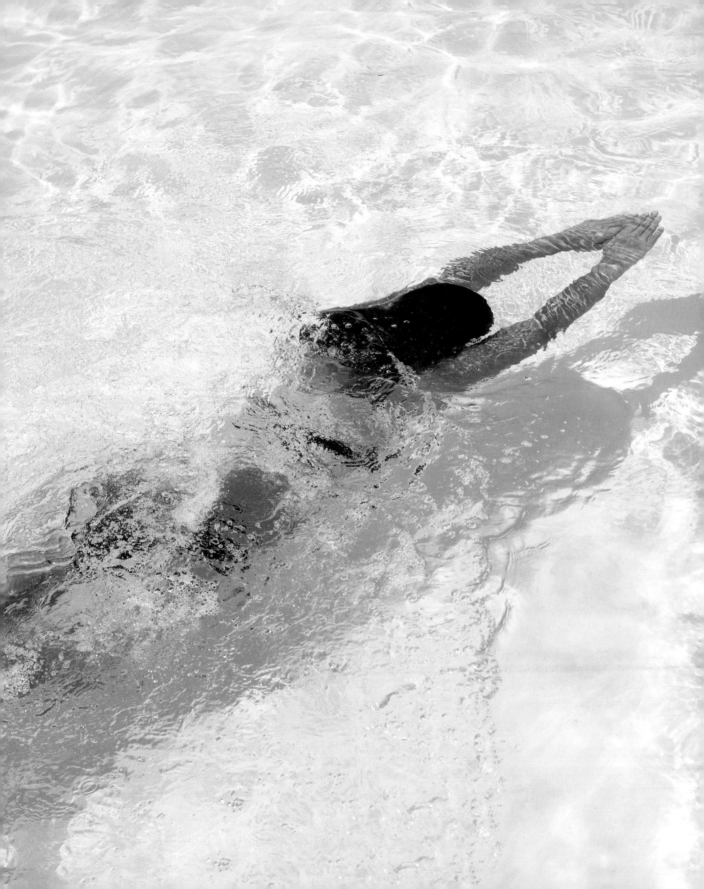

the full-strength program day four

Daily menu

- **Breakfast: Cinnamon Toast (see page 164). Chopped banana**

- **Morning snack: Red Delicious apple or a handful of black grapes**

- **Lunch: Potato Salad (see right). Cottage cheese with dates and pistachios. Bowl of mixed red salad leaves with Pecan Oil and Red Wine Vinegar Dressing (see page 168). "High-ORAC" fruit (see page 49)**

- **Afternoon snack: handful of walnuts**

- **Dinner: broiled eggplant, red onion, zucchini, and red, green, and yellow bell peppers brushed with olive oil and sprinkled with Mexican Hot Chili Sauce (see page 169). Red Lentil Dhal (see page 170). Mashed sweet potato. Purple sprouting broccoli. About 1½ ounces bittersweet chocolate and/or a handful of raspberries**

- **Drinks: 2½ cups lowfat or nonfat milk. Unlimited tea (including herbal or fruit tea) and mineral water. Glass of pomegranate, blueberry, cranberry, or apple juice**

- **Supplements: see page 145**

To make the potato salad for lunchtime, boil chopped Russet potatoes with the skins on. When cool, mix them with chopped red onion and lowfat mayonnaise. When you broil the red peppers and cook the dhal for dinner, make extra for tomorrow's lunch.

Daily exercise routine

Go for a walk, cycle, or swim (see pages 144–145). Do the stretch exercises from days one to three, then add the following leg stretch.

Leg stretch

1 Stand with your left side near a wall, your left hand on the wall.
2 Bend your left knee slightly, then bend your right leg behind you and grasp your right ankle with your right hand. Keep your knees facing forward (don't twist them). Ease your foot toward your bottom. Hold for a count of five. Turn around, and repeat on the other side.

Acupressure

Stimulate the acupoints from previous days, then work on Stomach 36, also known as St36, *ZuSanLi*, or Leg Three Miles.

The right walking stick

If you use a walking stick, select one with a T-shaped handle, which offers better support than a crook shape. Check it's the correct height by standing up straight with your usual walking shoes on and your arms at your sides. The top of the stick should reach the crease on the underside of your wrist. This allows your elbow to flex to 15 to 20 degrees when you hold the stick while standing.

Stomach 36

1 Locate the point four fingerwidths below your kneecap to the outside of the shinbone in a hollow that forms when you bend your knee, between the shin bone and the leg muscle.
2 Gradually build up the pressure on the acupoint and then gradually release it. Do this for about one minute, while breathing slowly and deeply. Now repeat on the other leg.

day five

Daily menu

- **Breakfast: Apple and Raspberry Smoothie (see page 166)**

- **Morning snack: Red Delicious apple or a handful of black grapes**

- **Lunch: Kidney Bean, Beet, and Feta Salad (see page 166). Cold broiled red pepper drizzled with olive oil. Cold red lentil dhal. Wholewheat bread roll (optional). "High-ORAC" fruit (see page 49)**

- **Afternoon snack: handful of pecans**

- **Dinner: Mango Salsa Salmon Steaks (see page 171). Broccoli. Green peas. Baked Russet potato. Baked or stewed apple with vanilla-flavored yogurt with live cultures**

- **Drinks: 2½ cups lowfat or nonfat milk. Unlimited tea (including herbal or fruit tea) and mineral water. Glass of pomegranate, blueberry, cranberry, or apple juice**

- **Supplements: see page 145**

Make a pot of green tea this evening and put some prunes in the liquid while still hot. Leave the prunes to soak overnight, ready for tomorrow's breakfast.

Daily exercise routine

Walk, swim, or cycle (see pages 144–145). Do the first four exercises of the program followed by the wall sits below.

Wall sits

1 Stand with your back a little way away from a wall, your feet hip-width apart, and your toes pointing forward. Lean back and press your lower back into the wall. Pull in your abdominals, relax your shoulders, and bend your knees and hips to about 90 degrees.

2 Hold this position for as long as is comfortable—at least 10 seconds at first, building up to one minute eventually.

Acupressure

Today's point is used specifically to treat arthritis of the knee joint. It's called Stomach 35, St35, *DuBi*, or Calf's Nose. Stimulate this point after you've worked on the acupoints on days one to four.

Stomach 35

1 This point is located just below the knee. To find it, bend your knee and search with your fingers in the outside dimple of your knee joint, below the kneecap on the outside of the ligament.

2 Press lightly, then slowly increase the pressure to the limit of comfort. Release the pressure gradually and build it up again to stimulate the point. Continue pressing for about one minute, while breathing slowly and deeply. Repeat on the other side.

the full-strength program day six

Daily menu

- **Breakfast: prunes soaked overnight in green tea, sprinkled with pistachio nuts**

- **Morning snack: Red Delicious apple or a handful of black grapes**

- **Lunch: slice of ham, cheese, or smoked salmon. Spiced Lentil Salad (see page 168). Bowl of mixed red salad leaves with Pecan Oil and Red Wine Vinegar Dressing (see page 168). "High-ORAC" fruit (see page 49)**

- **Afternoon snack: handful of walnuts**

- **Dinner: broiled boneless, skinless chicken breast halved first marinated in olive oil, garlic, and herbs. Green beans. Saffron Rice (see page 170). Blueberry and Cranberry Mold (see page 173)**

- **Drinks: 2½ cups lowfat or nonfat milk. Unlimited tea (including herbal or fruit tea) and mineral water. Glass of pomegranate, blueberry, cranberry, or apple juice**

- **Supplements: see page 145**

Today, I show you the last acupressure point in the sequence of six. From today, check the acupressure points you've used during this program on a daily basis. Continue to massage those that are still tender.

Daily exercise routine

Continue to walk, cycle, or swim, as outlined on pages 144–145. Do the stretches from the previous days, then add these mini squats.

Mini squats

1 Stand with your hands on your hips, your feet 3 feet apart, and your toes turned out. Bend your knees, and, keeping your knees turned out over your toes, squat down as low as you can—don't lean forward.

2 Lift up and down using slow movements. Do this 10 times initially, and work up to 20.

Acupressure

The final acupressure point I'd like to introduce to you is Triple Heater 6, also known as SJ6, *ZhiGou,* or Branch Ditch. It's used to dispel stagnant qi in the upper body, and to treat shoulder and back pain.

Triple heater 6

1 You can find this point four finger widths above your wrist on the back of your forearm, between your two lower arm bones.

2 Press lightly on this point, and gradually increase the pressure as much as you can tolerate. Release the pressure gradually and build it up again to stimulate the point. Continue this for about one minute, while breathing slowly and deeply. Repeat on the other side.

Sitting comfortably

If you can, buy an adjustable chair—it will support your back and prevent pain. When sitting, move your hips back as far as you can until they are against the back of the chair. Next, adjust the seat height until your feet are flat on the floor. Your hips should be at the same height or slightly higher than your knees. Adjust the backrest, if possible, so it is comfortably resting in the curve of your lower back.

day seven

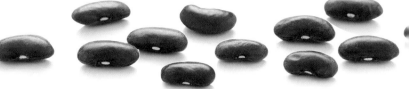

Daily menu

- **Breakfast: Apple, Kiwi, and Blueberry Smoothie (see page 166)**

- **Morning snack: Red Delicious apple or a handful of black grapes**

- **Lunch: Salmon and Mixed Bean Lunch Bowl (see page 168). Speciality bread, such as sun-dried tomato bread or garlic and herb bread. "High-ORAC" fruit (see page 49)**

- **Afternoon snack: handful of pecans**

- **Dinner: Extra-Spicy Chili Beans (see page 172). Tortilla chips. Mashed avocado (mixed with lemon or lime juice and crème fraîche or sour cream). Mexican Hot Chili Sauce (see page 169). Chocolate, Prune, and Pecan Squares (see page 173)**

- **Drinks: 2½ cups lowfat or nonfat milk. Unlimited tea (including herbal or fruit tea) and mineral water. Glass of pomegranate, blueberry, cranberry, or apple juice**

- **Supplements: see page 145**

Daily exercise routine

Keep up your walking, cycling, or swimming routine (see pages 144–145). Do the stretch exercises from days one to six followed by these calf stretches.

Calf stretches

1 Stand comfortably with your feet slightly apart. With your right foot, step forward so your left heel comes off the ground.

2 Bend your right knee a little and place both hands on your right thigh. Slowly, press your left heel back toward the ground so you feel your left calf stretching. Hold the stretch for a count of five. Repeat the stretch on your right leg.

Consulting an acupuncturist

Having followed the full-strength program for one week, you should have noticed an improvement in your arthritis symptoms. It's now time to consult a complementary therapist for individual advice. I suggest you have a course of traditional Chinese acupuncture to complement the acupressure techniques you have been using. Acupuncture can regulate the flow of qi energy in your body to help reduce joint pain and inflammation, and it can improve your range of movement.

During a consultation, the practitioner will ask you about your medical history and examine you physically, which might include an assessment of your tongue and pulse (see page 42). Sterile, disposable, slender needles are inserted into the skin at selected acupoints (this is usually painless, but you can notice a slight pricking, tingling, or buzzing sensation). An acupuncturist will use between six and 12 needles, usually on points on the hands and feet. He or she might stimulate the needles with a small, low-frequency electrical current or with a burning herb called moxa. (This technique is called moxibustion.) Some needles are left in position for a few seconds, while others might be left 30 minutes or longer. A course of 12 treatments over six weeks, can significantly improve your arthritis symptoms. To find an accredited acupuncturist, go to page 174.

the full-strength program day eight

Daily menu

- **Breakfast: toast with a scraping of olive-oil spread. Berry and Apple Jelly (see page 165)**

- **Morning snack: Red Delicious apple or a handful of black grapes**

- **Lunch: ½ sliced red bell pepper. Bowl of mixed bean salad (canned or homemade). Rye bread. Bowl of mixed red salad leaves with Pecan Oil and Red Wine Vinegar Dressing (see page 168). "High ORAC" fruit (see page 49)**

- **Afternoon snack: handful of walnuts**

- **Dinner: broiled fish fillet with Chili Fries (see the box on the right). Corn. Peas. About 1½ ounces bittersweet chocolate and/or a handful of cherries**

- **Drinks: 2½ cups lowfat or nonfat milk. Unlimited tea (including herbal or fruit tea) and mineral water. Glass of pomegranate, blueberry, cranberry, or apple juice**

- **Supplements: see page 145**

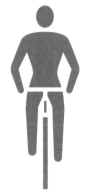

Over the next few days I suggest several different complementary therapies that are beneficial for arthritis. Once you' find a therapy that suits you, find ways to incorporate it into your life.

Daily exercise routine

Go walking, cycling, or swimming (see pages 144–145). Do your usual sequence of stretches (see days one to seven) followed by today's stretch.

Horizontal forward bends

1. Sit on the floor on a comfortable surface, such as an exercise mat. Keep your legs together and to the front.
2. Reach forward and try to touch your toes (or as far down your legs as you can manage). Hold the stretch for a count of 10.

Magnetic patches

Today, I'd like you to buy adhesive magnetic patches and stick two or three on tender points around your most painful joints to improve circulation and promote healing. (Magnetic patches are increasingly used to boost healing of bone fractures.) You might also like to try placing a patch over the Governing Vessel 14 acupoint (see page 147). Keep the patches in place for five days, remove them for two days and then reapply.

Chili fries

To make the Chili Fries for today's dinner, cut four to six Russet potatoes into big, chunky fries, leaving the skins on. Coat them in chili oil (simply mix 4 tablespoons olive oil with 2 teaspoons cayenne pepper). Bake the fries in a heated 400°F oven 25 minutes, or until tender and golden. This makes enough fries to serve four.

day nine

Daily menu

- **Breakfast: Apple and Carrot Breakfast Muffins (see page 164)**

- **Morning snack: Red Delicious apple or a handful of black grapes**

- **Lunch: Borscht Soup (see page 166). Wholewheat bread roll (optional). "High-ORAC" fruit (see page 49)**

- **Afternoon snack: handful of pecans**

- **Dinner: Beef, Black Bean, and Chilli Stir-Fry (see page 169). Mexican Hot Chili Sauce, optional (see page 169). Noodles. Lowfat vanilla ice-cream with Blueberry and Cranberry Mold (see page 173)**

- **Drinks: 2½ cups lowfat or nonfat milk. Unlimited tea (including herbal or fruit tea) and mineral water. Glass of pomegranate, blueberry, cranberry, or apple juice**

- **Supplements: see page 145**

Daily exercise routine

Go for a walk, cycle, or swim today as outlined on pages 144–145. Add today's hamstring stretches to the sequence you've learned so far on the program.

Hamstring stretches

1 Sit on the floor on a comfortable surface, such as an exercise mat, with your legs straight and spread apart.

2 Bend your right knee out to the side and bring your right foot up against your left knee. Try to keep your right knee in contact with the ground. Keeping your left leg straight, slowly bend forward, and try to touch your left ankle or foot. Hold the stretch for a count of 10. Repeat with the other leg.

Aromatherapy

Today's complementary technique uses a blend of essential oils that, when massaged into painful joints, can significantly decrease arthritis pain. As described on page 27, add the following oils to 100 ml carrier oil: eight drops each of eucalyptus and lavender oils; four drops each of marjoram, peppermint, and rosemary oils. Gently massage this oil blend into painful joints daily from now on.

Using a keyboard

When using a keyboard, your shoulders should be relaxed, your upper arms vertical, your forearms horizontal, and your wrists in a neutral, balanced position, not cocked upward. Ergonomically designed keyboards with specifically shaped key pads and integral wrist rests are available. I think it's worth investing in one. Also, use a document holder to minimize neck movement.

the full-strength program day ten

Daily menu

- **Breakfast: Omelet with Caramelized Sweet Potato and Red Onions (see page 165)**

- **Morning snack: Red Delicious apple or a handful of black grapes**

- **Lunch: Smoked Peppered Mackerel and Beet Salad (see page 168). Wholewheat bread roll (optional). "High-ORAC" fruit (see page 49).**

- **Afternoon snack: handful of walnuts**

- **Dinner: Eggplant and Potato Curry (see page 170). Mexican Hot Chili Sauce, optional (see page 169). Turmeric and Almond Rice (see page 170). Four large black or red plums**

- **Drinks: 2½ cups lowfat or nonfat milk. Unlimited tea (including herbal or fruit tea) and mineral water. Glass of pomegranate, blueberry, cranberry, or apple juice**

- **Supplements: see page 145**

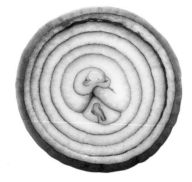

Daily exercise routine

Do the nine stretches you've learned so far, followed by today's stretch. Walk, cycle, or swim as described on pages 144–145.

Lower back strengtheners

1 Lie on a comfortable but firm surface, such as an exercise mat. Bend your knees, place your feet flat on the floor, and put your hands behind your head.

2 Now contract the muscles of your lower abdomen and buttocks, so your pelvis tilts upward and the small of your back flattens against the floor.

3 Hold this stretch for a count of five, then relax and repeat five to 10 times.

Herbalism

Today, I'd like you to start using a herbal medicine to ease your arthritis symptoms. The herb I've selected as most appropriate for the full-strength program is extract of rosehips, which can significantly reduce the pain and stiffness associated with all types of arthritis. You can buy it from healthfood stores. Check it's likely to suit you by reading about it on page 28. Start taking a supplement that supplies the equivalent of at least 2,000 mg (2 g) whole rosehip. Take it once or twice a day, depending on the severity of your joint pain and stiffness.

Prolonged squatting

Squatting for long periods can increase the risk of developing knee osteoarthritis, and can exacerbate symptoms if you already have it. Avoid squatting during activities such as gardening. (If you kneel instead, always use a padded kneeler or strap-on knee pads.)

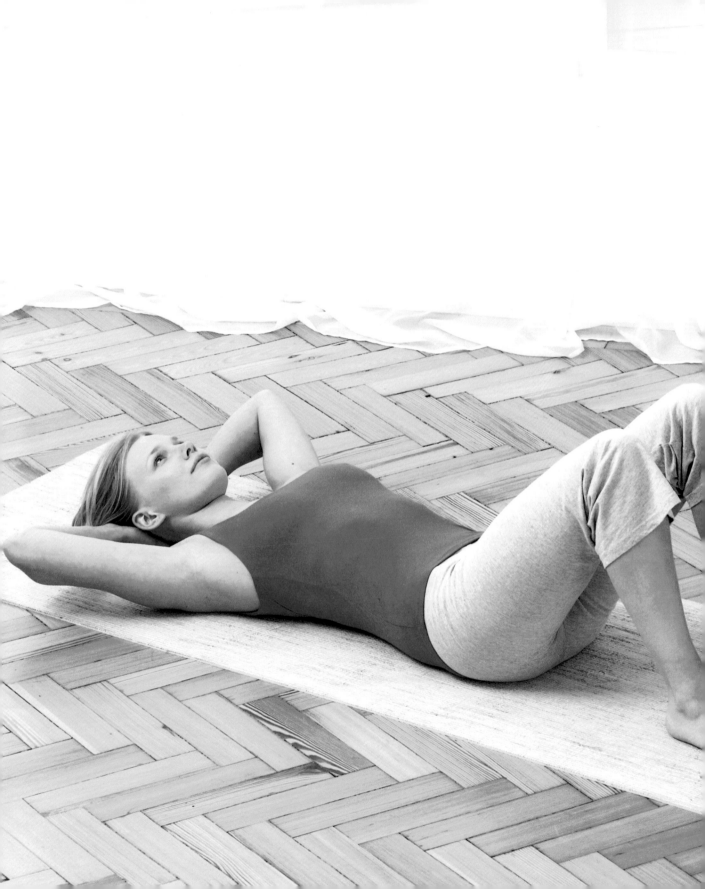

the full-strength program day eleven

Daily menu

- **Breakfast: Cinnamon Toast (see page 164)**

- **Morning snack: Red Delicious apple or a handful of black grapes**

- **Lunch: sliced avocado, beefsteak tomato, and mozzarella cheese arranged on a bed of mixed red salad leaves drizzled with Pecan Oil and Red Wine Vinegar Dressing (see page 168). Wholewheat bread roll. "High-ORAC" fruit (see page 49)**

- **Afternoon snack: handful of pecans**

- **Dinner: Baked Whole Fish with Lemon and Herbs (see page 137, moderate program). Baked Russet potato. Bowl of mixed red salad leaves drizzled with Pecan Oil and Red Wine Vinegar Dressing (see page 168). Chilled Strawberry Soup (see page 172)**

- **Drinks: 2½ cups lowfat or nonfat milk. Unlimited tea (including herbal or fruit tea) and mineral water. Glass of pomegranate, blueberry, cranberry, or apple juice**

- **Supplements: see page 145**

This evening, put some prunes in green tea and soak them overnight for tomorrow's breakfast.

Daily exercise routine

Continue with your walking, cycling, or swimming routine as described on pages 144–145. Do the stretches from days one to 10, then add these leg lifts.

Leg lifts 1

1 Lie on your back on a comfortable but firm surface, with your knees bent and your feet flat against the floor. Bring your right knee to your chest.

2 Return your leg to its starting position, then let it lie on the floor, shaking it gently to relax the muscles. Repeat step one, this time raising your left leg.

Chakra meditation

This chakra meditation draws healing energy up through your body's seven energy centers (see page 44), which are each associated with a particular color. Today, I'd like you to focus on opening each chakra in turn by spending two minutes visualizing the color associated with it.

Correct lifting

Never bend and lift at the same time. Instead, follow these guidelines for safe lifting techniques.

- Stand close to the load. Position your feet on each side of it.
- Squat down by bending at the knees and hips.
- Grasp the object with both hands (not fingers) and keep your elbows tucked in.
- Lean forward slightly and, in one smooth action, straighten your hips and knees while lifting the object (keep it close). To lower an object, do these steps in reverse. Always keep your back straight and don't twist.

Start with your base chakra and the color red. Work up to your crown chakra and the color white. Imagine your crown chakra is expanding and giving out a white light that envelops your body in a sphere of healing energy. Visualize this becoming concentrated within your most painful joints.

day twelve

Daily menu

- **Breakfast: prunes soaked in green tea (from day eleven)**
- **Morning snack: Red Delicious apple or a handful of black grapes**
- **Lunch: Kidney Bean, Beet, and Feta Salad (see page 166). Wholewheat bread roll (optional). "High-ORAC" fruit (see page 49)**
- **Afternoon snack: handful of walnuts**
- **Dinner: Hungarian Goulash (see page 171). Mexican Hot Chili Sauce, optional (see page 169). Red or brown rice. About 1½ ounces bittersweet chocolate and/or a handful of raspberries**
- **Drinks: 2½ cups lowfat or nonfat milk. Unlimited tea (including herbal or fruit tea) and mineral water. Glass of pomegranate, blueberry, cranberry, or apple juice**
- **Supplements: see page 145**

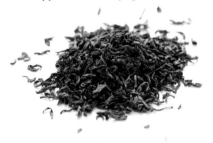

Cook extra rice for your dinner today to eat it in a salad for tomorrow's lunch.

Daily exercise routine

Go walking, cycling, or swimming (see pages 144–145). Do the stretch exercises from days one to eleven, followed by these leg lifts.

Leg lifts 2

1 After you've done yesterday's leg lifts, straighten your right leg and lift it as high as you can off the ground.
2 Lower your right leg slowly and relax. Repeat with your left leg. Repeat this five to 10 times on each side.

Copper therapy

Today, I'd like you to start using a pair of Copper Heelers (shoe inserts; see page 33). These are available from drug stores, or from www.theoriginalcopperheeler. com. Alternatively, if you haven't already used a copper bracelet (as suggested on day nine of the moderate program), start using one now. If you're already using a copper bracelet, put one on the other arm, too.

Hot chili peppers

The heat of chili peppers is rated using the Scoville scale—consult it whenever you're choosing a chili for a recipe. The hotter the pepper, the more it will help your arthritis.

- Pure capsaicin: 15,000,000–16,000,000
- Habanero: 350,000–577,000
- Scotch Bonnet: 100,000–350,000
- Jamaican hot pepper: 100,000–200,000
- Thai pepper: 50,000–100,000
- Cayenne pepper, Tabasco pepper: 30,000–50,000
- Serrano pepper: 10,000–23,000
- Tabasco sauce: 7,000–8,000
- Wax pepper: 5,000–10,000
- Jalapeño pepper: 2,500–8,000
- Rocotillo pepper: 1,500–2,500
- Poblano pepper: 1,000–1,500
- Anaheim pepper: 500–1,000
- Pimento and pepperoncini: 100–500

the full-strength program day thirteen

Daily menu

- **Breakfast: Apple, Kiwi, and Blueberry Smoothie (see page 166)**

- **Morning snack: Red Delicious apple or a handful of black grapes**

- **Lunch: Spiced Lentil Salad (see page 168). Canned tuna mixed with chopped tomato, parsley, and lowfat mayonnaise. Bowl of red salad leaves drizzled with Pecan Oil and Red Wine Vinegar Dressing (see page 168). Focaccia. "High-ORAC" fruit (see page 49)**

- **Afternoon snack: handful of pecans**

- **Dinner: pasta with red pesto. Chopped tomato and red onion. Bowl of mixed red salad leaves drizzled with Macadamia Nut and Lemon Juice Dressing (see page 137) and sprinkled with Parmesan shavings and mixed seeds. Peach Melba with Pecans (see page 172)**

- **Drinks: 2½ cups lowfat or nonfat milk. Unlimited tea (including herbal or fruit tea) and mineral water. Glass of pomegranate, blueberry, cranberry, or apple juice**

- **Supplements: see page 145**

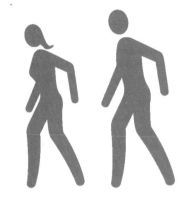

Daily exercise routine

Keep up your walking, cycling, or swimming regime, as outlined on pages 144–145. Remember to warm up and cool down first. Do the stretch exercises from the previous days, followed by these pelvic circles.

Pelvic circles

1 Lie on your back on a comfortable but firm surface, such as an exercise mat. Hug your knees in to your chest with a hand on each knee.

2 Keep your feet and knees together and draw circles in the air with your knees (near to your chest). Do 10 circles in one direction, then 10 in the opposite direction.

Mud bath

Today, I'd like you to use some Dead Sea mineral mud (available from drug stores and online) in the bath. Run a deep bath hot enough to make the bathroom steamy. Massage the thick, black mud into your most painful joints and add any excess to the bath water. Get into the bath and soak for at least 20 minutes in the mineral-rich water. Rinse off in a shower. If you want, you can reapply the black mineral mud to your most painful joints, then wrap a bandage around each joint and leave on as a healing poultice up to 24 hours.

Keep moving
Muscles and joints need oxygen to retain their flexibility. When they stay in the same position for a length of time they become fatigued and lacking in oxygen, and this triggers pain. Take regular movement breaks at least every 10 to 15 minutes to help maintain muscle and joint mobility.

day fourteen

Daily menu

- **Breakfast: high-fiber cereal and lowfat or nonfat milk sprinkled with fresh blueberries**

- **Morning snack: Red Delicious apple or a handful of black grapes**

- **Lunch: ½ avocado with shrimp and chopped cilantro leaves. Red salad leaves with Pecan Oil and Red Wine Vinegar Dressing (see page 168). Focaccia or garlic and herb bread. "High ORAC" fruit (see page 49)**

- **Afternoon snack: handful of walnuts**

- **Dinner: Salmon with Pink Peppercorns and Red Lentils (see page 171). Mashed Russet potatoes. Bowl of mixed red leaves with Pecan Oil and Red Wine Vinegar Dressing (see page 168). Stewed apples and raspberries**

- **Drinks: 2½ cups lowfat or nonfat milk. Unlimited tea (including herbal or fruit tea) and mineral water. Glass of pomegranate, blueberry, cranberry, or apple juice**

- **Supplements: see page 145**

Daily exercise routine

Keep up your walking, cycling, or swimming routine, as described on pages 144–145. Do the stretch exercises from days one to thirteen, then add the following hip circles.

Hip circles

1 Lie on your back in the same starting position as step one of yesterday's pelvic circles.

2 Keeping your feet together, make circles with your knees. Each knee should go in the opposite direction to the other and as wide as possible to the side before coming back in to complete each circle. Do 10 circles like this, then reverse direction and do another 10 with each knee circling in the opposite direction.

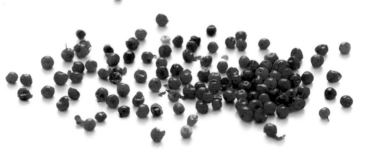

Consulting a Reiki master

Having followed the full-strength plan for two weeks, it's now time to consult a holistic practitioner, and I suggest you experience spiritual healing with a Reiki master. Reiki healing channels universal energy through the chakra centers on which you meditated on day eleven. A treatment session lasts about an hour, during which you lie clothed on a table. The practitioner holds his or her hands on or over your body in 12 basic positions for five minutes each: four of these are on your head, four on the front of your body, and four on the back. You might feel heat emanating from the healer's hands. You can feel relaxed or sometimes invigorated after a Reiki session. To find a practitioner, see the resources on page 175.

continuing the full-strength program

Well done—you have followed the full-strength program for 14 days. Now I'd like you to repeat the program so it lasts for a full 28 days. Eating a diet so high in antioxidants (20,000 ORAC units a day or more) should significantly ease your arthritis symptoms. If this is the case, apply the principles of the program every day from now on.

If the full-strength program doesn't provide symptom relief, and you've already tried the previous programs, it's likely that some other component of your diet, apart from an imbalance between omega-6s and omega-3s or exposure to nightshade plants, is affecting your joint symptoms. You might want to try excluding meat from your diet (see pages 51–52), or acid-forming foods (see pages 52–53), or to follow a full elimination-and-challenge diet. An elimination-and-challenge diet involves excluding foods to which you suspect you might have an intolerance. In surveys, the foods most likely to provoke arthritis symptoms are: bacon, beef, caffeine, corn, dairy products, grapefruit, lamb, lemons, malt, oranges, pork, rye, sugar, tomatoes, wheat, and yeast. You might want to exclude all these from your diet to see if your symptoms improve. You can then reintroduce eliminated foods one by one, usually at three-day intervals, to see if they provoke symptoms. Here's how a suspect food is typically reintroduced:

- Day 1
  Breakfast: eat a small quantity of test food, such as 1 ounce cheese. Monitor for adverse reactions over four hours. If OK:

  Lunch: eat twice the amount eaten that morning, in other words, 2 ounces. Monitor for adverse reactions over 4 hours. If OK:
  Dinner: eat twice the amount eaten at lunch, in other words 4 ounces cheese.
- Day 2
  Eat a basic elimination diet, consisting of foods you know don't upset your symptoms. Avoid the test food. Monitor for delayed reactions to the test food.
- Day 3
  Assess whether or not your symptoms are worse as a result of eating the test food. If an adverse reaction occurs, continue to avoid the test food and wait 48 hours after all symptoms have gone before testing another food. If the results are unclear, repeat the steps from day one, but using larger amounts of the suspect food. If the suspect food does not worsen your symptoms, add it to the list of foods you can eat. Start testing a new food on day four using the same method.

Although you can try this on your own at home, it's best to follow a full elimination-and-challenge diet under the supervision of a naturopath or nutritionist who is experienced in diagnosing food intolerances. Another approach to diagnosing food intolerances is to have a blood test that assesses the way your white blood cells react to a variety of different food extracts, or to measure your levels of IgG anti-food antibodies. These tests (see page 50) are at least 70 percent effective in pinpointing culprit foods.

Your long-term diet

If you stay on the full-strength program, continue to eat lots of fresh fruit and vegetables, selected nuts, and oily fish to maximize your intake of anti-inflammatory antioxidants. Go back and re-read pages 47–49—about the high-ORAC diet—to refresh your memory of the highest scoring fruit and vegetables.

Recipes Continue to explore recipes containing high antioxidant foods, especially fish-based and vegetarian recipes. You will find some recipe suggestions at www.naturalhealthguru.co.uk, and you can post your own favorites there, too, for other followers of the full-strength program to try.

Your long-term supplement regime

Continue taking the recommended supplements for the full-strength program (see page 145) long term. Research supports their use at this high level for significant beneficial effects on joint health. If, up until now, you have taken only the supplements in the recommended list, you might also want to add in one or more of the supplements in the optional list for extra benefit. Alternatively, if your arthritis is well controlled, you can reduce the dose of your supplements back down to the levels suggested in the moderate program and see if this lower dose remains beneficial.

Your exercise routine

After performing the full-strength exercises for four weeks, you should notice an improvement in muscle strength and joint flexibility. Continue doing these stretch and range-of-motion exercises, ideally twice a day. Also try to fit in some walking, cycling, or swimming. Over time, extend your aerobic exercise sessions to 30 to 40 minutes on most days of the week. Consider starting other activities, such as dancing, gardening, bowling, or golfing, too.

Diagnostic techniques for food intolerance

There is little evidence to support the use of VEGA electrodermal testing, applied kinesiology (muscle strength) testing, or hair mineral analysis, and I don't personally recommend these. Having said that, a few people have undoubtedly found them helpful.

Your therapy program

The full-strength program has shown you how to use acupressure to ease your joint symptoms, and has introduced you to several other complementary techniques, including aromatherapy, magnetic patches, copper, Dead Sea mineral mud, herbal medicine, and meditation. Continue using the therapies you find beneficial, and continue to consult the acupuncturist and Reiki healer I suggested you see on days seven and fourteen if you found their treatments helpful. You might also want to explore some of the other therapies I mentioned in Part Two, such as chiropractic or osteopathy.

Monitoring your joint symptoms

From now on, I suggest you continue monitoring and scoring your joint symptoms at least once a month, to make sure you continue to show some benefits. If your joint scores stop showing an improvement, or if they start to worsen again, check you are taking the level of supplements I recommend as desirable for the full-strength program and consider taking one or more of those I give as options for additional health benefits (see page 145). If your joint symptoms still remain troublesome, I suggest you visit a naturopath or nutritionist for individually tailored advice about your diet.

breakfast recipes

apple and carrot breakfast muffins

. . . .

serves 4

²/₃ cup mixed, dried fruit, such as
    blueberries, cranberries, raisins,
    chopped prunes, and chopped dates
1 cup pecans, chopped
½ cup plus 1 tablespoon wholewheat
    flour
1 cup old-fashioned rolled oats
¹/₃ cup dried skim milk powder
1½ tablespoons baking powder
1 tablespoon ground cinnamon
1 tablespoon ground ginger
2 omega-3-enriched eggs, lightly beaten
½ cup olive oil
3 tablespoons honey
3 tablespoons maple syrup
1 tablespoon vanilla extract
1 large Red Delicious apple, grated
1 cup peeled and grated carrots

1   Heat the oven to 350°F.
2   Mix together the dried fruit,
    pecans, flour, rolled oats,
    milk powder, baking powder,
    cinnamon, and ginger in a bowl.
3   In a separate bowl, beat
    together the eggs, oil, honey,
    maple syrup, and vanilla
    extract. Add the apple and
    carrot, and then the flour
    mixture from the first bowl.
4   Mix briefly with a large spoon.
    Spoon into 8 large muffin paper
    cases, and bake 20 minutes.
    Serve warm or allow to cool.

cinnamon toast

. . . .

serves 4

4 slices wholewheat bread
1 tablespoon ground cinnamon
1 tablespoon soft light brown or
    granulated sugar
3 tablespoons butter

1   Heat the broiler to low. Toast
    the bread on one side under
    the broiler. Mix together the
    cinnamon, sugar, and butter.
2   Butter the untoasted side, then
    place back under the broiler
    until evenly brown. Cut into
    fingers and serve hot.

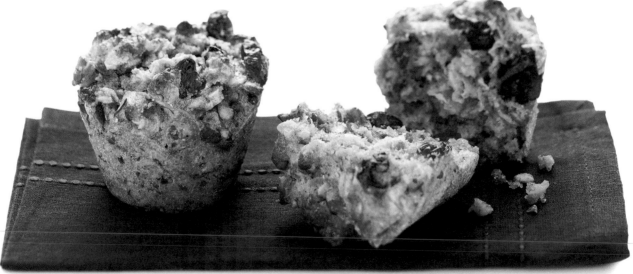

berry and apple jelly

makes three ½-pint jars

7 cups fresh berries, such as
   raspberries, strawberries,
   blueberries, or blackberries, rinsed
3 Red Delicious apples, chopped
   (including skin, core, and seeds)
Juice and seeds of 2 lemons
About 3¼ cups sugar

1 Heat the oven to 350°F.
   Sterilize three ½-pint canning
   jars and lids by heating them in
   the oven for 15 minutes.
2 Put all the fruit, juice, and
   seeds in a stainless-steel
   preserving pan. Add enough
   water to cover the fruit and
   cook on the stovetop until the
   mixture is soft. Pour into a
   cheesecloth bag and hang over
   a nonmetallic bowl overnight,
   to catch the juice (or pass
   through a conical sieve).
3 Pour the juice into a measuring
   jug and record the volume. For
   every 2½ cups juice you need
   to add 2 cups sugar.
4 Put the juices and sugar in

a clean jam pan and heat gently
to dissolve the sugar. Boil
rapidly until the jelly reaches
setting point (220°F). Remove
from the heat and skim off any
froth, then pour into the jars
and seal with lids. Process in a
water bath. Label and store in a
cool, dry, place.

omelet with caramelized sweet potato and red onions

serves 4

2 tablespoons olive oil
1 red onion, thinly sliced
1 sweet potato, peeled and grated
1 garlic clove, chopped
1 sprig oregano, leaves chopped
1 tablespoon maple syrup or honey
8 omega-3-enriched eggs
1 handful grated cheese, such as
   cheddar, mozzarella, or Gruyère
Freshly ground black pepper

1 Heat half of the olive oil in a
   saucepan and sauté the onion,
   sweet potato, garlic, and
   oregano. Add the maple syrup
   or honey and cook 2 minutes
   longer, stirrring.
2 Beat the eggs lightly and
   season with black pepper.
   Heat the remaining olive oil in
   an omelet pan over high heat.
   Tip in the eggs, cook until
   there's only a little runny
   egg left, then remove from
   the heat.
3 Sprinkle the sweet potato
   and onion over one half of
   the omelet. Add the cheese
   and season with black pepper.
4 Return to the heat 30 seconds.
   Flip the uncovered side of the
   omelet over, slide onto a plate,
   and serve.

left: apple and carrot breakfast muffins

apple, kiwi, and blueberry smoothie

. . . .

serves 4

4 red eating apples, cored
4 kiwifruit, peeled
2 cups blueberries
Scant ½ cup unsweetened apple juice

1 Whiz the fruit in a blender
then stir in the apple juice
slowly (using more or less
juice to create the consistency
you like).

apple and raspberry smoothie

. . . .

serves 4

4 Red Delicious apples, cored
2 cups raspberries
Scant ½ cup unsweetened apple juice

1 Whiz the fruit in a blender
then stir in the apple juice
slowly (using more or less
juice to create the consistency
you like).

lunch recipes

kidney bean, beet, and feta salad

. . . .

serves 4

2 cups cooked or cooked canned kidney
   beans
1 raw or cooked beet, peeled and grated
1 carrot, peeled and grated
1 red onion, chopped
4 tomatoes, chopped
²/₃ cup crumbled feta cheese
1 red lettuce, such as lollo rosso or red
   oak leaf, chopped

For the dressing:
4 tablespoons walnut oil
1 garlic clove, crushed
1 tablespoon red wine vinegar
1 handful herbs, such as basil and
   parsley, chopped
Freshly ground black pepper

1 Put the dressing ingredients in
a small jar with a screwtop lid
and shake.
2 Mix the salad ingredients
together and pour the dressing
over the top. Toss and serve.

borscht soup

. . . .

serves 4

1 tablespoon olive oil
1 red onion, chopped
1 garlic clove, crushed
1 large celery stick, chopped
1 small fennel bulb, chopped
5 beets, peeled and grated
2½ cups vegetable stock or water
2 tomatoes, skinned
1 handful baby spinach leaves
Grated zest and juice of 1 unwaxed
   lemon
1 tablespoon chopped basil
4 tablespoon crème fraîche or plain
   yogurt with live cultures
Freshly ground black pepper

1 Heat the olive oil in a pan and
sauté the onion, garlic, celery,
and fennel 10 minutes. Add
the beet and cover with the
stock. Simmer 5 minutes,
then add the tomatoes and
cook 5 minutes longer. Add
the spinach leaves and lemon
zest and juice and cook 2
minutes longer.
2 Puree in a blender until smooth.
Season with plenty of black
pepper. Serve hot or cold in
four bowls with a sprinkling of
basil and a tablespoon of crème
fraîche or yogurt in each.

right: borscht soup

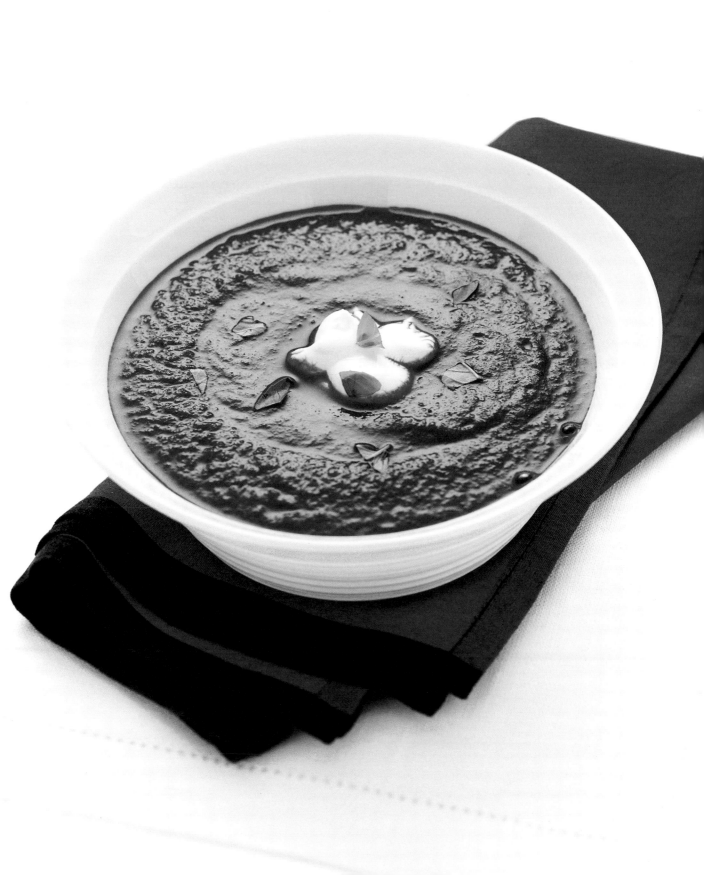

salmon and mixed bean lunch bowl

serves 4

4 Russet potatoes
1 red lettuce, for example, lollo rosso or red oak leaf, shredded
3 cups mixed cooked beans, such as red kidney beans, chickpeas, or black beans
14 ounces cold, cooked salmon (poached, broiled, or roasted), flaked
1 red onion, chopped
1 slice red cabbage, shredded
½ cucumber, chopped
1 handful cherry tomatoes
1 handful chopped parsley

For the dressing:
4 tablespoons walnut oil
1 garlic clove, crushed
1 tablespoon red wine vinegar
1 tablespoon herbs, such as parsley or cilantro, chopped
Freshly ground black pepper

1 Boil the potatoes in their skins until cooked. Leave to cool until warm and chop into chunks.

2 Put the dressing ingredients in a screwtop jar and shake. Mix together all the salad ingredients and pour the dressing over the top. Toss and serve immediately.

pecan oil and red wine vinegar dressing

serves 4

6 tablespoons pecan oil
2 tablespoon red wine vinegar, or raspberry vinegar
Freshly ground black pepper

1 Put the ingredients in a screwtop jar and shake. Store the dressing in a cool, dry place, where it will keep for several days.

spiced lentil salad

serves 4

1 cup red lentils
1 red onion, finely chopped
2 garlic cloves, crushed
1-inch piece gingerroot, peeled and finely chopped
1 tablespoon cumin seeds, crushed
1 tablespoon coriander seeds, crushed
4 tablespoons extra virgin olive oil
1 large carrot, grated
Grated zest and juice of 1 unwaxed lemon
1 handful cilantro leaves, chopped
4 hearts of lettuce
Freshly ground black pepper

1 Simmer the lentils in 2½ cups water for minutes, or according to package directions, until tender. Drain.

2 Sauté the onion, garlic, ginger, cumin, and coriander seeds in olive oil. Add the spiced onion mixture, carrot, and lemon zest and juice to the lentils. Stir.

3 Season with black pepper and sprinkle with cilantro leaves. Serve warm or chilled on top of the lettuce leaves.

smoked peppered mackerel and beet salad

serves 4

¾ cup topped and tailed green beans
1 red lettuce, shredded
1 small beet, peeled and grated
Grated zest and juice of 1 unwaxed lemon
2 tablespoons olive oil
4 fillets smoked mackerel with black peppercorns

For the dressing:
4 tablespoons lowfat yogurt
2 tablespoons honey
1 tablespoon wholegrain mustard
1 handful dill, chopped

1 Blanch the green beans in boiling water 1 minute. Drain, refresh under cold running water, and dry.

2 Put the dressing ingredients in a screwtop jar and shake.

3 Toss the lettuce, beet, and beans with the lemon zest and juice and olive oil. Divide between 4 plates and put a mackerel fillet on top of each. Pour the dressing over the top.

dinner recipes

mexican hot chili sauce

serves 4

2 tablespoons extra virgin olive oil
1 red onion, finely chopped
1 tablespoon ground cumin
2 garlic cloves, crushed
2 carrots, grated
1 handful chopped oregano
4 hot red chilies (habaneros),
    seeded and finely chopped
Grated zest and juice of 2 limes
2 tablespoons red wine vinegar

1 Heat the oil in a pan and sauté
   the onion, cumin, and garlic
   until the onions are soft. Add
   the carrots, 1 cup water, and
   oregano and bring to a boil.
   Simmer slowly until the
   carrots are tender.
2 Add the chilies, lime
   zest and juice, and
   vinegar. Puree in a
   blender until smooth.

beef, black bean, and chili stir-fry

serves 4

1 pound beef tenderloin, cut into strips
2 red onions, thinly sliced
2 garlic cloves, chopped
1 red chili, finely chopped
2 tablespoons extra virgin olive oil
1 bag (10-oz.) baby spinach leaves,
    washed and shaken dry
1 head of broccoli, cut into florets
1 green bell pepper, seeded and
    chopped
½ cucumber, cut into thin strips
7 ounces black bean sauce

1 Stir-fry the beef, onions, garlic,
   and chili in olive oil until brown.
   Add the spinach, broccoli,
   green pepper, and cucumber
   and stir-fry 3 minutes longer.
2 Stir in the bean sauce, heat
   through for 1 minute and serve.

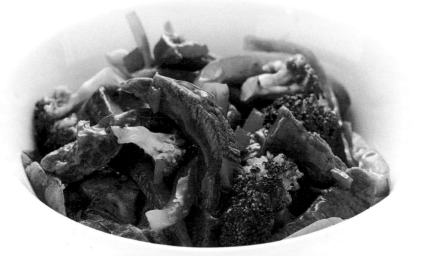

beef, black bean, and chili stir-fry

red lentil dhal

· ·

serves 4

1 cup red lentils, washed
4 tablespoons olive oil
1 red onion, chopped
1 garlic clove, crushed
1 tablespoon coriander seeds, ground
1 tablespoon ground cumin
1 tablespoon turmeric
1 tablespoon fenugreek seeds, ground
1 tablespoon cayenne pepper
1-inch piece gingerroot, peeled and
   grated
4 tablespoons red wine vinegar
1 handful cilantro leaves, chopped

1 Cook the lentils in 2½ cups
   water, or according to the
   package directions. Drain,
   retaining the cooking liquid.
2 Heat the oil in a pan and sauté
   the onion and garlic until they
   start to color.
3 Mix together the spices and
   red wine vinegar to make a
   thick paste. Add the spice
   paste to the onion mixture and
   slowly sauté 5 minutes. Add
   the drained lentils, cilantro, and
   some of the cooking liquid to
   obtain your preferred thickness.

eggplant and potato curry

· ·

serves 4

2 tablespoons cumin seeds
2 tablespoons mustard seeds
4 tablespoons olive oil
2 red onions, chopped
3¾ cups cubed eggplants
¼ cup red lentils
1 cup vegetable stock
1 tablespoon turmeric
1 tablespoon shredded coconut
2 green chilies, slit lengthwise
1-inch piece gingerroot, peeled and
   finely chopped
1 tablespoon cayenne pepper
2 tablespoons ground coriander
1 handful cilantro leaves, chopped

1 Sauté the cumin and mustard
   seeds in the oil until they start
   to crackle. Add the onions and
   stir-fry until soft.
2 Add all the remaining
   ingredients, cover, and simmer
   15 to 20 minutes until all the
   vegetables are tender. Stir
   occasionally and, if the curry
   becomes too dry, add more
   water. Serve sprinkled with the
   cilantro leaves.

turmeric and almond rice

· ·

serves 4

1 heaped cup long-grain rice, such as
   basmati
2 tablespoons turmeric
1¼ cups coconut milk
1 large handful slivered almonds
1 handful parsley or cilantro leaves,
   chopped

1 Boil the rice in 2 cups water,
   then simmer gently until all the
   water is absorbed.
2 Add the turmeric to the coconut
   milk and stir well before pouring
   over the rice.
3 Simmer the rice until the milk is
   absorbed. Put on a serving dish,
   add the slivered almonds and
   fluff with a fork. Serve sprinkled
   with parsley or cilantro.

saffron rice

· ·

serves 4

1 large pinch saffron stamens
4 tablespoons olive oil
4 cups boiling stock
1 large red onion, chopped
2 garlic cloves, crushed
2 pieces cinnamon stick
4 whole cloves
10 cardamom pods, seeds only
1¾ cups long-grain rice
1 handful parsley or cilantro leaves,
   chopped

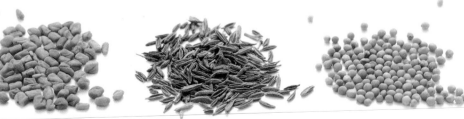

1 Cover the saffron with 3 tablespoons boiling stock and leave to soak 10 minutes.

2 Heat the oil in the pan and sauté the onions, garlic, cinnamon, cloves, and cardamom seeds. Add the rice and stir 5 minutes.

3 Add the remaining stock and bring to a boil. Add the saffron and its water. Cover and simmer 25 minutes. Drain and sprinkle with parsley or cilantro.

mango salsa salmon steaks

serves 4

4 salmon fillets
1 tablespoon olive oil

For the salsa:
1 mango, seeded and flesh finely chopped
1 Red Delicious apple, finely chopped with skin on
Grated zest and juice of 1 unwaxed lime
1 red chili, seeded and finely chopped
1 handful cilantro leaves, chopped

1 Mix the salsa ingredients and marinate in the refrigerator at least 1 hour.

2 Brush the salmon fillets with olive oil and broil until the flesh flakes easily. Serve the salmon steaks with the mango salsa on the side.

salmon with pink peppercorns and red lentils

serves 4

4 salmon fillets
3 tablespoons extra virgin olive oil
1 cup red lentils, rinsed
2 red onions, chopped
1 garlic clove, crushed
2 tablespoons pink peppercorns
1 tablespoon crème fraîche or sour cream
1 handful basil leaves, chopped
Freshly ground black pepper

1 Heat the oven to 325°F.

2 Put the salmon in a baking dish, drizzle with 1 tablespoon of olive oil, and season well with black pepper. Cover with aluminim foil and roast 15 minutes, or until the flesh flakes easily.

3 Meanwhile, cook the red lentils in 2½ cups water, or according to the package directions. Heat 1 tablespoon of olive oil in a pan and sauté the red onion and garlic until just soft.

4 Stir in the pink peppercorns, crème fraîche or sour cream, and basil. Drain the lentils and toss in 1 tablespoon of olive oil. Divide between 4 plates. Put a piece of salmon on top of each and spoon the sauce over.

hungarian goulash

serves 4

1 tablespoon olive oil
3 red onions, chopped
2 garlic cloves, crushed
1 green bell pepper, seeded and chopped
1 red bell pepper, seeded and chopped
1 pound lean stewing steak, cut into small chunks
1 tablespoon sweet paprika
2 tablespoons hot paprika
4 tomatoes, chopped
2 tablespoons tomato paste
2 bay leaves
2/3 cup vegetable stock or water
2/3 cup red wine
3 unpeeled Russet potatoes, cubed
Grated zest and juice of 1 unwaxed lemon
Freshly ground black pepper

1 Heat the oven to 300°F.

2 Heat the olive oil in a pan and sauté the onions, garlic, and peppers until the onions are golden. Add the meat and cook 5 minutes, stirring. Stir in the paprikas, tomatoes, tomato paste, bay leaves, stock, and red wine.

3 Transfer to a baking dish with a lid, cover, and cook 2 hours. Add the potatoes and lemon zest and juice and cook an hour longer, or until the meat and potatoes are tender. Season well with black pepper.

extra-spicy chili beans

serves 4

1¼ cups dried kidney beans, soaked
    overnight and rinsed
1 tablespoon virgin olive oil
2 red onions, chopped
4 garlic cloves, crushed
4 carrots, peeled and grated
2 red bell peppers, seeded and chopped
2 celery sticks, finely chopped
2 tablespoons ground cumin
6 tablespoons ground coriander
2 red chilies, chopped
8 ripe tomatoes, chopped
2 tablespoon tomato paste
²/₃ cup red wine
Grated zest and juice of 1 unwaxed
    lemon
¹/₃ cup bulgur wheat
1 handful chopped cilantro leaves
Freshly ground black pepper

1 Simmer the beans in 5 cups
    water 60 minutes; strain and
    retain the cooking liquid.
2 Heat the oil in a pan and sauté
    the red onions and garlic,
    then add the carrots, peppers,
    celery, beans, and spices and
    sauté 5 minutes.
3 Add the tomatoes and paste,
    red wine, lemon zest and juice,
    bulgur wheat, and about 2½
    cups of the retained liquid.
    Cover and simmer 40 minutes.
4 Add the cilantro leaves and
    extra liquid (if necessary).
    Cover and simmer 20 minutes
    longer. Season with black
    pepper and serve.

dessert recipes

fresh strawberry coulis

serves 4

1½ pints strawberries, hulled and
    halved
1 tablespoon confectioners' sugar
Lowfat vanilla ice cream, to serve

1 Put the ingredients in a metal
    bowl, add 2 tablespoons water,
    and cover. Place over a pan of
    simmering water 90 minutes,
    then strain the juice. Serve with
    the ice cream.

chilled strawberry soup

serves 4

1½ pints strawberries, hulled and
    halved
1 tablespoon sugar
½ cup light red wine, such as Beaujolais
Grated zest and juice of 2 oranges
Grated zest and juice of 1 unwaxed
    lemon
Freshly ground black pepper

1 Put the strawberries in a bowl
    (reserving a few) and sprinkle
    with the sugar and a little black
    pepper. Leave to marinate.
2 Pour the wine into a pan, add
    both zests, the lemon juice and
    half the orange juice, then bring

to a boil. Simmer, uncovered,
until the volume reduces by
half. Strain and leave to cool.
3 Stir the wine into the
    strawberries and add the
    remaining orange juice. Whiz
    in a blender. Season with black
    pepper and serve with the
    reserved strawberries.

peach melba with pecans

serves 4

Scant ½ cup sugar
1 vanilla bean, or 2 tablespoons vanilla
    extract
4 peaches, peeled and halved
1¾ cups raspberries
½ cup confectioners' sugar
1 handful pecans, chopped

1 Put the sugar, vanilla bean, and
    1¼ cups water in a pan and
    simmer, stirring, until the sugar
    dissolves. Poach the peaches
    in the syrup 5 minutes.
2 Whiz the raspberries and
    confectioners' sugar in a
    blender. Add a little water (or
    syrup) to make a coulis. Serve
    the cool peaches with the
    coulis. Sprinkle with pecans.

right: blueberry and cranberry mold

chocolate, prune, and pecan squares

● ●

serves 8

2 ounces bittersweet chocolate (at least 70 percent cocoa solids)
1 tablespoon butter
¼ cup semidried prunes, chopped and soaked overnight in black or green tea
½ cup pecans, chopped
2 omega-3-enriched eggs
Scant 1 cup packed soft light brown sugar
Scant ½ cup self-rising flour

1　Heat the oven to 350°F.
2　Melt the chocolate and butter in a metal bowl over simmering water. Remove from heat and stir in all the remaining ingredients.
3　Pour into a 10- x 16-inch baking pan lined with parchment paper. Bake 30 minutes. Cool on a wire rack and cut into squares.

blueberry and cranberry mold

● ●

serves 4

1 cup blueberries, fresh or thawed from frozen
2 cups cranberry juice
1 envelope unflavored gelatin
4 handfuls fresh mixed berries, for example, strawberries, and raspberries

1　Put the blueberries and half the cranberry juice in a saucepan and bring to a boil. Simmer gently 2 minutes.
2　Heat the rest of the cranberry juice until it bubbles, then sprinkle in the gelatin stirring, until it dissolves. Pour into the blueberry mixture and mix well.
3　Rinse out a mold with cold water, then pour in the gelatin mixture. Leave to cool, stirring occasionally. Place in the refrigerator to set.
4　To turn out the gelatin mold, dip the mold in hot water, invert onto a plate, and tap the bottom. Serve with mixed berries piled in the middle.

resources

Visit www.naturalhealthguru.co.uk for more information, medical references and to post comments and questions about the programs.

Arthritis
- American Arthritis Society
  www.americanarthritis.org
- American College of Rheumatology
  www.rheumatology.org
- Arthritis Foundation
  www.arthritis.org
- Arthritis Insight
  www.arthritisinsight.org
- Arthritis Society of Canada
  www.arthritis.ca
- Canadian Arthritis Network
  www.arthritisnetwork.ca

Complementary medicine associations
- Alternativemedicinecare.net
  www.alternativemedicinecare.net
- American Holistic Medical Association
  www.holisticmedicine.org
- National Center for Complementary and Alternative Medicine (NCCAM)
  www.nccam.nih.gov
- The Ontario Society of Physicians for Complementary Medicine
  www.ospcm.org

Acupuncture
- American Association of Acupuncture and Oriental Medicine
  www.aaaomonline.org
- American Academy of Medical Acupuncture
  www.medicalacupuncture.org
- Canadian Association of Acupuncture & Traditional Chinese Medicine
  www.caatcm.com

Aromatherapy
- Canadian Federation of Aromatherapists (CFA)
  www.cfacanada.com
- National Association for Holistic Aromatherapy (NAHA)
  www.naha.org

Chiropractic and osteopathy
- American Chiropractic Association (ACA)
  www.amerchiro.org
- American Osteopathic Association
  www.osteopathic.org
- Canadian Chiropractic Association
  www.ccahiro.org
- Canadian Osteopathic Association
  www.osteopathic.ca

Food intolerance
- American Academy of Allergy Asthma & Immunology
  www.aaaai.org
- Canadian Society of Allergy and Clinical Immunology
  www.csaci.medical.org
- World Allergy Organization
  www.worldallergy.org

Herbal medicine

- International Register of Consultant Herbalists and Homeopaths
  www.irch.org
- American Herbalist Guild
  www.americanherbalistguild.com
- Ontario Herbalists Association
  www.herbalists.on.ca

Homeopathy

- American Institute of Homeopathy
  www.homeopathyusa.org
- Canadian National United Professional Association of Trained Homeopaths
  www.nupath.org
- North American Society of Homeopaths
  www.homeopathy.org

Massage

- American Massage Therapy Alliance
  www.amtamassage.org
- Canadian Massage Therapy Association
  www.cmta.ca

Naturopathy

- American Association of Naturopathic Physicians
  www.naturopathic.org
- American Naturopathic Medical Association
  www.anma.com
- Canadian Association of Naturopathic Doctors (CAND)
  www.cand.ca
- Canadian Association of Naturopathic Medicine
  www.ccnm.edu

Qigong

- Qigong Association of America
  www.qi.org
- Qigong Association of Canada
  www.canadaqigong.org

Quitting smoking

- The Foundation for a Smoke-free America
  www.anti-smoking.org
- Action on Smoking and Health US
  www.ash.org
- Action on Smoking and Health Canada
  www.ash.ca

Reflexology

- Reflexology Association of America
  www.reflexology-usa.org
- Reflexology Association of Canada
  www.reflexologycanada.ca

Reiki

- The Reiki Alliance
  www.reikialliance.com
- Canadian Reiki Association
  www.reiki.ca

Yoga

- American Yoga Association
  www.americanyogaassociation.org
- Canadian Yoga Alliance
  www.canadianyogicalliance.com
- Canadian Yoga Association
  www.canadianyogaassociation.com

index

acknowledgments

The publisher would like to thank the following photographic libraries for permission to reproduce their material. Every care has been taken to trace copyright holders. However, if we have omitted anyone, we apologize and will, if informed, make corrections to any future edition.

page 85 Takeshi Niguchi/Amana Images/Getty Images; **91** John-Francis Bourke/Zefa/Corbis; **121** Jukka Rapo/ Gorilla Creative Images/Getty Images; **125** David Lees/ Iconica/Getty Images; **149** ICHIRO/Japan Taxi/Getty Images; **157** DBP

Height and weight chart on page 71 © Crown copyright material is reproduced with the permission of the Controller of HMSO and Queen's Printer for Scotland.

Author's acknowledgments

I would like to thank my husband, Richard, who willingly provided invaluable back-up and support during those long hours of research and writing. I would also like to thank everyone who has helped in bringing this book to fruition, including Grace Cheetham at Duncan Baird, Judy Barratt and Kesta Desmond—who insured consistency throughout —and, of course, my inimitable agent, Mandy Little.